A CRITICAL APPROACH TO SURROGACY

This comprehensive text makes an important contribution to the study of surrogacy, developing a novel theoretical framework through which to understand the broader social contexts as well as individual decisions at play within surrogacy arrangements.

Drawing on empirical research conducted by the authors and supplemented by secondary analyses of media, legislative and public accounts of surrogacy, the book engages with the key stakeholders involved in the practice of surrogacy. Specifically, it canvases the standpoints of women who act as surrogates, intending parents who commission surrogacy arrangements, children born through surrogacy, clinics that facilitate the arrangements, and politicians and journalists who engage with the topic.

Through a focus on capitalism as a means of orientating ourselves to the topic of surrogacy, the book highlights the vulnerabilities that potentially arise in the context of surrogacy, as well as the claims to agency invoked by some parties in order to mitigate vulnerability. In so doing, the book demonstrates that the psychology of surrogacy must be broadly understood as an orientation to particular ways of thinking about children, reproduction and economies of labour.

Dr Damien W. Riggs is an Associate Professor in Social Work at Flinders University and an Australian Research Council Future Fellow.

Dr Clemence Due is a Senior Lecturer in the School of Psychology at the University of Adelaide, Australia.

Critical Approaches To Health

Series Editors: Kerry Chamberlain and Antonia Lyons

The Routledge *Critical Approaches to Health* series aims to present critical, inter-disciplinary books around psychological, social and cultural issues related to health. Each volume in the series provides a critical approach to a particular issue or important topic, and is of interest and relevance to students and practitioners across the social sciences. The series is produced in association with the International Society of Critical Health Psychology (ISCHP).

Titles in the series:

Urban Poverty and Health Inequalities
A Relational Approach
Darrin Hodgetts and Ottilie Stolte

Constructing Pain
Historical, Psychological and Critical Perspectives
Robert Kugelmann

Digital Health
Critical and Cross-Disciplinary Perspectives
Deborah Lupton

A Critical Approach to Surrogacy
Reproductive Desires and Demands
Damien W. Riggs and Clemence Due

A CRITICAL APPROACH TO SURROGACY

Reproductive Desires and Demands

Damien W. Riggs and Clemence Due

Routledge
Taylor & Francis Group
LONDON AND NEW YORK

ISCHP
International Society of Critical Health Psychology

First published 2018
by Routledge
2 Park Square, Milton Park, Abingdon, Oxon OX14 4RN

and by Routledge
711 Third Avenue, New York, NY 10017

Routledge is an imprint of the Taylor & Francis Group, an informa business

British Library Cataloguing in Publication Data
A catalogue record for this book is available from the British Library

Library of Congress Cataloging in Publication Data
Names: Riggs, Damien W., author. | Due, Clemence, author.
Title: A critical approach to surrogacy : reproductive desires and demands / Damien W. Riggs, Clemence Due.
Description: 1 Edition. | New York : Routledge, [2018] | Series: Critical approaches to health | Includes bibliographical references and index.
Identifiers: LCCN 2017017358| ISBN 9781138123618 (hb : alk. paper) | ISBN 9781138123656 (pb : alk. paper) | ISBN 9781315648750 (ebk)
Subjects: LCSH: Surrogate motherhood. | Human reproduction. | Parenthood. | Capitalism.
Classification: LCC HQ759.5 .R54 2017 | DDC 306.874/3–dc23
LC record available at https://lccn.loc.gov/2017017358

ISBN: 978-1-138-12361-8 (hbk)
ISBN: 978-1-138-12365-6 (pbk)
ISBN: 978-1-315-64875-0 (ebk)

Typeset in Bembo
by Wearset Ltd, Boldon, Tyne and Wear

Damien and Clemmi would like to dedicate this book to Joplin. We didn't know you very long, but we are thankful for all of the joy you brought into our lives.

CONTENTS

SERIES EDITOR PREFACE

Critical Approaches to Health

Health is a major issue for people all around the world, and is fundamental to individual wellbeing, personal achievements and satisfaction, as well as to families, communities and societies. It is also embedded in social notions of participation and citizenship. Much has been written about health, from a variety of perspectives and disciplines, but a lot of this writing takes a biomedical and causally positivist approach to health matters, neglecting the historical, social and cultural contexts and environments within which health is experienced, understood and practised. It is an appropriate time to introduce a new series of books that offer critical, social science perspectives on important health topics.

The *Critical Approaches to Health* series aims to provide new critical writing on health by presenting critical, interdisciplinary and theoretical writing about health, where matters of health are framed quite broadly. The series will include books that range across important health matters, including general health-related issues (such as gender and media), major social issues for health (such as medicalization, obesity and palliative care), particular health concerns (such as pain, doctor–patient interaction, health services and health technologies), particular health problems (such as diabetes, autoimmune disease and medically unexplained illness), or health for specific groups of people (such as the health of migrants, the homeless and the aged), or combinations of these.

The series seeks above all to promote critical thought about health matters. By critical, we mean going beyond the critique of the topic and work in the field, to more general considerations of power and benefit, and, in particular, to addressing concerns about whose understandings and interests are upheld and whose are marginalized by the approaches, findings and practices in these various domains of health. Such critical agendas involve reflections on what constitutes knowledge, how it is created and how it is used. Accordingly, critical approaches consider epistemological and theoretical positioning, as well as issues of methodology and practice, and seek to examine how health is enmeshed within broader social relations and structures. Books within this series take up this challenge and seek to provide new insights and understandings by applying a critical agenda to their topics.

In the current book, Damien W. Riggs and Clemence Due take up the complex issues involved in surrogacy. They show how the ways that we orient to surrogacy are shaped by normalized views within the world, including the view that to be a good citizen is to reproduce. They argue convincingly that this is not an automatic or 'natural' view, but one that is made to appear natural. Through these expectations and norms, surrogacy becomes a viable (and indeed sensible) orientation for those who (for whatever reason) are unable to have genetically related children. Riggs and Due situate their work within broad historical and social forces, demonstrating how capitalism, and especially neoliberalism, enable and shape current understandings of surrogacy. They argue that capitalism is central to valuing reproduction and the desire to have genetically related children. Within the current social order surrogacy becomes one way of achieving this, where the bodies of certain women are treated as objects of labour for consumers, a process often reframed as engaging in natural practices of womanhood.

A central tenet within this book is a focus on vulnerability, across all aspects of surrogacy. Framed through capitalism, the authors highlight how people become vulnerable due to the 'drive to (re)produce'. This produces reproductive vulnerability for intending parents who have experienced medical or social infertility in a world in which genetic relationships are privileged. In commissioning surrogacy arrangements, intending parents mitigate their potential vulnerability by emphasizing their agency, making decisions and determining their futures (to lay claim to genetic contributions to a child), and hence creating a competent self. Women who act as surrogates are also rendered vulnerable due to their social positioning, their potential for exploitation and commodification, and the possible negative health implications involved. Riggs and Due acknowledge and discuss the tensions across these vulnerabilities.

In developing their arguments throughout the book, Riggs and Due disrupt dominant ideas around surrogacy as a normalized form of reproduction. Their critical perspectives allow for interrogations around how to move beyond capitalist approaches to surrogacy. They conclude the book by examining such possibilities, including considering how individuals function within broader global contexts, the ethics of surrogacy and the potential for creating opportunities to promote health equity and wellbeing for all actors engaged in surrogacy arrangements.

We welcome this substantial contribution to the *Critical Approaches to Health* series, offering timely coverage of an important field which has far-reaching implications for our understandings of the nature of kinship and relationships, and what this means for health and wellbeing.

Antonia Lyons and Kerry Chamberlain
April 2017

ACKNOWLEDGEMENTS

We begin by acknowledging the sovereignty of the Kaurna people, the First Nations people upon whose land we live in Adelaide, South Australia.

We would like to thank Antonia Lyons and Kerry Chamberlain, series editors, for believing in this book from the beginning. We would also like to thank Russell George, Elizabeth Rankin and their team at Taylor & Francis for making this such an enjoyable publishing experience. Thanks must also go to the people who so kindly shared their experiences with us as we have sought to grapple with the topic of surrogacy.

Damien would like to thank Clemmi for a decade of friendship, collegiality and camaraderie. The thoughts and reflections in this book represent the culmination of many years of conversations, concerns and writing that we have undertaken together, made always enjoyable by the context of our friendship, despite the challenges of the topic. Other colleagues and friends have also contributed to my thinking about surrogacy, including Donna McCormack, Sophie de Rohan, Deborah Dempsey and Elizabeth Peel. Some of the ideas presented in this book were honed through engagement from audiences at the Queer Kinship and Relationships conference held in Poland in 2015, the Con/Tested conference at Cambridge University in 2014, a Feast Festival forum in Adelaide in 2014, an invited seminar given at Stockholm University in 2014 organized by Johanna Gonduin, and an Australian Critical Race and Whiteness Studies conference held in Adelaide in 2012.

Clemmi would like to thank Damien for many years of thoughtful discussion and a safe space in which to explore ideas and develop her thinking in relation to all aspects of parenting (including practical ones!). The many, many conversations we have had together have helped me consider surrogacy and parenting more broadly in all its nuances, and in ways I would never have done without our long and wonderful conversations. My work in this area is also framed by conversations concerning health equity and social determinants of health with Anna Ziersch and others in the Southgate team. As I write this, my partner, Braden, is caring for our two sick children, so thanks also go to him for practical help and listening to me bounce ideas around.

Aspects of the analysis reported in Chapter 4 were originally published as Riggs, D. W. and Dempsey, D. (2015). Gay men's narratives of pregnancy in the context of commercial surrogacy. In N. Burton (Ed.), *Birth and its meanings: Representations of pregnancy, childbirth and parenting*, and is reprinted here with permission from Demeter Press.

Aspects of the analysis reported in Chapter 6 were originally published as Riggs, D. W. and Due, C. (2016). Constructions of gay men's reproductive desires on surrogacy clinic websites. In M. Davies (Ed.), *Babies for sale? Transnational surrogacy, human rights and the politics of reproduction*, and is reprinted here with permission from Zed Books.

1

BECOMING (DIS)ORIENTED

Faced with the topic of surrogacy, we are required to make a decision. The call to make a decision comes from many quarters: from the voices of women who act as surrogates, from feminist voices that have spoken both for and against surrogacy, from people who see surrogacy as their only route to becoming parents, from those whose religious affiliations lead them to hold a particular stance on the practice of surrogacy, from media representations of women who act as surrogates, from surrogacy agencies seeking to increase their revenue, and no doubt from many other quarters. Each of these calls to make a decision hails us in differing ways: as subjects expected to hold a moral position on surrogacy, as consumers, and as citizens invested in a particular relationship to the state. Yet, as can be seen in these differing calls, the possible decisions available to us are often competing, and difficult to encapsulate in one specific or consistent position.

Sara Ahmed's (2006) work on queer phenomenology provides us with one way through which we may map out a response to the multiple voices that shape contemporary understandings of surrogacy. Focusing on what it means to have an orientation, Ahmed suggests that one's orientation towards any given object or topic shapes and is shaped by how we inhabit the world around us. In order to see that we are indeed oriented in particular ways, however, first we must experience *dis*orientation. In other words, and as Ahmed suggests:

> We might think that we reach for whatever comes into view. And yet, what 'comes into' view, or what is within our horizon, is not a matter simply of what we find here or there, or even where we find ourselves as we move here or there. What is reachable is determined precisely by orientations that we have already taken.
>
> *(p. 55)*

To see one's own orientation towards any given topic, and particularly if one's orientation aligns with the dominant or normative orientation made intelligible by the world around us, is difficult precisely because it is often an orientation that we have taken implicitly, with little consideration of what that orientation brings. To see one's own orientation, then, requires us to fall from perspective, a perspective that for many of us is imbued with a claim that our own perspectives are 'normal', a 'given', and hence are taken for granted. To fall from perspective, as Fiona Nicoll (2000) suggests with regard to whiteness, is to acknowledge that the vantage point from which one is oriented is always partial, even if for (white, middle-class) people such as ourselves as the authors of this book, that partiality disappears through claims to the position of the universal subject.

For us, the topic of surrogacy – which we have written about for over half a decade – evokes multiple forms of disorientation, many of them induced by our explicit focus on the positions from which we speak, which bring together experiences of disadvantage and privilege. For Damien, as a parent to children with whom he does not share a genetic relationship, many of the narratives that circulate with regard to surrogacy are less than intelligible, and indeed can be marginalizing. As we shall see in the chapters to come, genetic relatedness is often (though not always) a valorized narrative amongst people who become parents through surrogacy. Also for Damien, a feminist critique of the commodification of women's bodies contributes to a sense of unease about the topic of surrogacy. Competing with these concerns, however, is a genuine respect for people's desire to have children, even if that desire may for many people be shaped by pronatalist discourses and the privileging of genetic relations. For Damien, then, the topic of surrogacy produces a disorientation that to date has stymied a desire to orient himself in ways that are respectful to all involved in the practice of surrogacy.

For Clemmi, the topic of surrogacy has similarly created disorientation. Clemmi is the mother of two children to whom she gave birth while in a heterosexual relationship with their father. As such, her family structure places her firmly within the norm concerning family. Clemmi's family structure therefore raises questions for her when engaging with any critique of the privileging of genetic relationships. That is, while she finds this aspect of many surrogacy discourses concerning, she also recognizes that – being a part of the 'norm' – it is important that she listens to the voices of others. However, as a full-time working mother, and a mother with experience of postnatal depression, Clemmi is also outside the norm of what is typically expected of mothers. This experience of being situated outside the norm of motherhood has meant that she has been able to interrogate discourses of 'good' mothering, which also come to the fore in relation to surrogacy – sometimes in relation to the intending parents, and sometimes in relation to the woman acting as a surrogate. As such, Clemmi also has found surrogacy to produce a disorientation around both family and parenting, and like Damien, she has struggled to find an orientation which will result in a respectful engagement with all those involved.

As two people who have thought long and hard about the topic of surrogacy, and thus for whom the topic is often salient, Ahmed's (2006) invitation to become disorientated has been useful in that it has led us to writing this book as a way to develop a mode of orientation that speaks to the many differing stakeholders invested in surrogacy. Albeit in highly differentiated ways, and as we shall see in the chapters to come, disorientation too shapes their entry into the world of surrogacy. The norm of reproductivity as a privileged mode of neoliberal citizenship, for example, potentially evokes disorientation for those who cannot (but wish to) fulfil the demand to genetically reproduce. For women who act as surrogates, the competing demands to provide for their children but gestate and hand over a child to other people potentially produces a disoriented relationship to norms of womanhood and motherhood. No doubt for many other stakeholders (including those whose primary focus is revenue), the competing demands of surrogacy – often framed within a binary of love or money – potentially produces other disorientations in relation to what it means to desire and to have a child.

For most of us, disorientation is not necessarily a desirable experience. As a counter to disorientation, most people are likely to seek ways to settle upon a way of being oriented. As we suggested above, writing this book is at least in part a means through which we may become oriented to the topic of surrogacy. For those who are disorientated by what is often framed as a 'failure' to reproduce, surrogacy may provide an orientation to reproductivity that affords them a claim to a place within the norm. For women who act as surrogates, the disorientation that may arise from the injunction to love *or* money is managed in complex (and often competing) ways that allow for an orientation to a morally defensible position, as we shall see below and further in Chapter 3.

Yet as Ahmed (2006) suggests in the quote above, the ways that we orient to particular objects are not accidental. Rather, they are shaped both by those orientations which are normalized or naturalized within the world around us, in addition to the orientations to which we then direct our attention. As we noted above, reproductivity is a norm to which neoliberal citizens are expected to orient, what Turner (2001) refers to as 'reproductive citizenship'. To be a good citizen is to reproduce, which requires an orientation to, or investment in, all that this entails. For many people this typically includes finding a partner with whom to have children, planning for a pregnancy, finding ways to achieve a pregnancy if this proves to be medically difficult (or is physically not possible if the couple are both cisgender and not heterosexual), and more broadly orienting one's life towards these goals. Whilst, as we will explore in greater detail below and in subsequent chapters, there is nothing natural or automatic about such an orientation, it is the fact that it is made to appear entirely natural and expected that forms one of the threads through which surrogacy becomes a viable orientation.

Another, and as we argue in this book, key, orientation that produces surrogacy as an intelligible means through which to have children is the logic of capitalism. It is common within writing on surrogacy to trace the practice of surrogacy back to biblical times (due to references made to surrogacy in the Bible). However, this, we feel, is something of a red herring, as it locates surrogacy within a very particular (altruistic, communal) understanding of the practice of women bearing children for others to raise. Certainly it could be argued that the trajectory through which surrogacy has become intelligible as a market commodity involves many orientations, some of which may be altruistic and premised upon caring relationships between or by women. This, however, is not the orientation that we believe dominates the field of surrogacy at present. Rather, and as we will argue in greater detail below, it is through a capitalist logic that surrogacy has become increasingly intelligible in modern societies.

Importantly, then, and following Jack Halberstam (2005), as we orient ourselves towards capitalism as a structuring logic of contemporary surrogacy practices, we must ultimately also seek to orient ourselves *away* from capitalism. This is not to suggest that, in unpacking what we see as the capitalist logic underpinning surrogacy, we can simply do away with capitalism. Rather, it is to suggest that our aim is not to deify capitalism as the only way to orient ourselves to the topic of surrogacy. Importantly, nor is it to replace a capitalism-focused account of surrogacy with one more akin to the biblical, altruistic, account mentioned above. Instead, by unpacking how capitalism frames both the desire to have genetically related children and surrogacy as one mode of achieving this, our aim is to create space for the possibility of other ways of thinking about citizenship – reproductive or otherwise. We explore this aim in greater detail in the final chapter of this book.

In what follows in this first chapter, we outline in further detail the orientation we propose with regard to the topic of surrogacy, acknowledging that it holds the potential to be disorienting, precisely for the ways in which it directs a magnifying glass at the operations of capital and fantasy that we suggest dually position surrogacy as intelligible within contemporary neoliberal contexts. Certainly, emphasising a capitalist logic is nothing new with regard to the topic of surrogacy. At the same time, however, there is a degree to which, at least in our reading, capitalism is often relegated to the sidelines of understandings of surrogacy practices, even when it is at the same time acknowledged as a driving force. It is perhaps unsurprising that this is the case, particularly since an emphasis on capitalism can both promote and undermine a particular position simultaneously (for example, capitalist arguments can be used to both validate and undermine the choices made by women who act as surrogates, or to validate and undermine the choices made by people who commission surrogacy arrangements).

We of course acknowledge that capitalism reproduces itself in nefarious ways, and that we are potentially complicit with this by endorsing an approach that orients itself towards capitalism. We are also mindful that having acknowledged the importance of falling from perspective, we are nonetheless advocating for a particular perspective on surrogacy (i.e. in taking up capitalism as a useful lens through which to consider surrogacy practices). Yet, as we will argue in this chapter and the one that follows, to state that capitalism is a structuring logic of surrogacy is not to make one singular claim. Rather – and where we think this book differs from those which have come before – we see capitalism as underpinning a diverse (and often competing) range of claims. Orienting ourselves to capitalism, then, is to consider the histories through which surrogacy comes to be rendered intelligible. In doing so, we aim to engage with some necessarily difficult questions concerning how the increasing number of surrogacy arrangements build upon ways of being oriented to oneself and to others that may in many ways be contrary to the desire to have a child 'of one's own'.

Notes on language

Before turning to the substantive aspects of this chapter, it is important for us to address the question of language with regard to surrogacy. Indeed, it could be argued that the language we use regarding surrogacy is constitutive of how we orient ourselves to the topic, and that in and of itself language is a substantive topic worthy of ongoing focus amongst those of us who study surrogacy. Certainly, those who have written on the topic previously have drawn attention to the fraught nature of the specific terms used. Over two decades ago Sharyn Roach Anleu (1992), and more latterly Marilyn Strathern (2003), have suggested that the word 'surrogate' itself is differentially used and understood. While commonly understood to refer to women who carry a baby for other people, Roach Anleu suggests that this is an incorrect use of the term, especially if the term 'mother' is appended to the word. Instead, Roach Anleu suggests instead that the correct use of the term 'surrogate mother' is in reference to a woman who commissions a surrogacy arrangement and intends to raise the child. Similarly, Helen Ragoné (1994) uses the term 'adoptive mother' to refer to women who commission surrogacy arrangements, although it should be noted that Ragoné's choice of language arose from the fact that at the time of her data collection surrogacy arrangements primarily involved women gestating children conceived from their own eggs, hence requiring that the intended mother adopt the child after they were born. Ragoné's use of the term 'adoptive mother' and Roach Anleu's use of the term surrogate mother to refer to women who commission a surrogacy arrangement align to a certain degree with the use of the term 'surrogate mother', both historically and still at times in the present, to refer to mothers who raise children who were not born to them (i.e. foster or adoptive mothers).

As Strathern (2003) argues, the reversal that has occurred (that is, from intended mothers being 'adoptive' or 'surrogate' mothers to women who gestate children for other people becoming known as 'surrogates') is embedded in at least two orientations to the topic of surrogacy. The first involves moves to disaggregate gestation from mothering. Whilst this move has not solely been taken up within feminist writing, feminist thought has certainly made a significant contribution to how we conceptualize motherhood. Such a contribution is of course important, given its role in deconstructing how motherhood is naturalized and taken as definitive of womanhood (Hays, 1996; Maushart, 1997). Yet as with any orientation, what has come with the denaturalization of motherhood from gestation is a potential devaluing of the intimate labour involved in gestation *itself*, a concern long raised by radical feminist voices who have opposed all forms of assisted reproductive technology (Cora, 1985).

The second orientation to surrogacy elaborated by Strathern (2003), which has led to the change in language described above, is the increased emphasis placed upon genetic relatedness as a key determinant of kinship. This is a topic that we will explore in further detail in Chapter 2, but suffice it to say here that with regard to the genetic relations between intended parents and the child being carried for them, this relationship is typically seen as more important than the biological relationship between the child and the woman who carries them. Even when both parents are not genetically related to the child, and as Charis Thompson (2005) has so eloquently demonstrated, claims to some form of genetic relatedness (and most certainly intent, which in some cases serves as a proxy for genetic relatedness, as we explore in detail below) are privileged over any claims the woman carrying the child may have.

While our discussion above is largely framed by research or theorising conducted within countries such as the United Kingdom and the United States, it is also important to consider the use of language in non-Western countries. In her research on surrogacy arrangements in Israel, for example, Elly Teman (2010) reports that a literal translation of the Hebrew word for 'surrogate' is 'inn keeper mother' (p. 21). Similarly, in her research on women who act as surrogates in India, Sharmilla Rudrappa reports that a literal translation of the Kannadese word for 'surrogate' is 'rental mother' (2015, p. 108). Whilst both of these terms retain the use of the word 'mother' (and certainly in both the United Kingdom and United States 'surrogate mother' would not be entirely atypical with reference to women who act as surrogates), the word is modified through the adjectives 'inn keeper' and 'rental'. Both these terms, we would suggest, are in many ways contrary to the word 'mother' and its normative disassociation from any notion of being temporary or receiving payment.

In addition to debates over how to refer to women who act as surrogates, recent discussions of surrogacy, specifically when such discussion involved intended parents from one country commissioning surrogacy arrangements in another country, have focused on how to describe this travel. As Inhorn and Patrizio (2012) note, such travel has alternately been described as a form of tourism (e.g. reproductive tourism, fertility tourism, procreative tourism), as travel (e.g. reproductive travel, fertility travel), or – most commonly – as 'cross-border reproductive care'. However, while being the most common term, Inhorn and Patrizio (2009) question the accuracy of 'cross-border reproductive care', which evokes an image of patients travelling for treatment – a situation which is not necessarily true of all those who travel. Consider, for example, a heterosexual couple, where the female partner has had a hysterectomy and the male partner produces viable sperm, and where both travel to engage surrogacy services. Which of these individuals is the patient? And if one or both of these individuals are positioned as the patient, what does this mean for the woman they may engage to act as a surrogate?

In contrast to the focus on describing cross-border travel, descriptors for those who undertake such travel are less frequently debated, though Inhorn and Patrizio

(2009) note that the term 'tourist' to refer to those who undertake cross-border travel may seriously overstate the 'pleasure' aspects of such travel. Beyond discussion of the appropriateness of the term 'tourist', those who undertake cross-border travel are most typically referred to simply by the reasons for their travel (e.g. 'people who undertake travel to access fertility services'). An exception to this is a term advocated for by Inhorn and Patrizio, namely 'reproductive exile'. This term, they suggest, better captures the experiences of their participants, who reported feeling '"forced" to leave their home countries to access safe, effective, affordable, and legal infertility care' (2009, p. 905). Other terms used to describe those who travel (or indeed those who do not) to undertake surrogacy arrangements are 'intending parents' and 'commissioning parents'.

Our orientation and use of language in this book will no doubt already be evident in what we have written above. As we will explore in more detail in the next section, we utilize the term 'intending parents' to centre how claims to intent function to authorize these parents as the only and indeed 'true' parents. Accompanying the term 'intending parents' within this book is the phrase 'women who act as surrogates', implied in which is the idea of 'women who provide a surrogate womb'. This is a contentious implication, given ongoing debates about the commodification of women's bodies, and the problems associated with disassociating gestation from women's sense of self and being. Aware of these contentions, we use the term advisedly, following two lines of thought. The first of these comes from the work of Teman (2010), in which she argues for the concept of 'body maps', through which women who act as surrogates partition out their wombs from the rest of their bodies so as to make some sort of peace with carrying a child for someone else. The second comes from the experiences of transgender men who bear children, and who are very much men engaging in this action, not women (Riggs, 2013, 2014).

Whilst we certainly do not wish to be complicit with the commodification of women's bodies, we believe that both of the lines of thought outlined above with regard to gestation and embodiment indicate the merits of thinking about surrogacy as something that women do as an action requiring the use of particularly focused parts of their body, even if such actions are rendered intelligible through very specific ways of thinking about women's bodies, reproductivity and capital. Finally, whilst aspects of this book focus on travel for the purposes of entering into surrogacy arrangements, there is no simple term that describes such travel given it cannot be abstracted from the broader logics that shape how travel is rendered intelligible in the context of securing a place within a norm of reproductive citizenship. This is not to say that travel is not our focus, but rather that with regards to terminology, it must be understood through reference to the broader logic of capitalism and intent.

Of course, it would be remiss of us if we did not attend to the word 'surrogacy' itself. Thus far in this chapter we have used the term without a clarifier such as 'commercial' or 'altruistic' or 'compensated'. We have done this purposively. Certainly, and as we will see in the chapters to come, there are differences between forms of surrogacy in terms of whether women who act as surrogates are paid or not. Yet as Roach Anleu (1992) points out, the distinction between 'altruistic' and 'commercial' surrogacy, much like the distinction between 'love' or 'money', elides the complex overlaps between the two (see also Zelizer, 2005). It elides them, we suggest along with authors such as Roach Anleu, precisely by ignoring the logic of capitalism underpinning reproduction more broadly, as we now explore in greater detail.

Reproduction and intentionality under capitalism

As we indicated above, capitalism is a central focus of this book. Following Ahmed's (2006) argument with regards to how we orient ourselves, any given orientation cannot be abstracted from the ways in which orientations are directed by broader social forces. Whilst, as we noted above, we do not wish to be seen as deifying capitalism, we believe it is vital to locate surrogacy within the context of capitalism, particularly the forms it takes under neoliberalism. More broadly than just surrogacy, of course, capitalism plays a central role in determining the value accorded to reproduction (Whittaker, 2015). The reproduction of human life is arguably a key logic of capitalism: humans are required for labour (even if some of that labour is apportioned to non-human animals or to non-sentient machines), and without humans there is no consumption of the labour and therefore no profit. Humans and their reproduction are thus central to capitalism (Sharp, 2000). Our concern in this section of the chapter, and in this book more broadly, however, is with how capitalism's aims are not per se to serve humanity. Rather, the purpose of capitalism is capital, which all too easily leads to the instrumentalization of humans, and – importantly – certain humans in particular.

A logic wherein the aims of capitalism are capital cannot, of course, be achieved without an investment in finding new ways to recruit labour forces and produce goods. Certainly, it is nothing new to make this point, as human bodies (as well as the bodies of other species, as we explore in greater detail in Chapter 2) have always been put to the service of producing goods. What differs with regard to surrogacy, and as Melinda Cooper and Catherine Waldby (2014) argue with regard to biomedical technologies more broadly, is that the human body becomes not simply a tool for enacting labour in order to produce goods, but rather the human body becomes a good in and of itself. Again, this claim is not new, and certainly others have likened surrogacy to either slavery or human trafficking (Allen, 1990; Das-Gupta & Das Dasgupta, 2014). Our argument here, however, is somewhat different, even if drawing upon these same logics.

In many ways, and as Ahmed (2006) again suggests, thinking about human bodies as themselves goods is part and parcel of a capitalist logic. What is specific about our claim here is the suggestion that what occurs in the treatment of women's bodies as goods in and of themselves is what Thompson (2005) in a somewhat different way has referred to as 'strategic naturalisation'. Much like the naturalization of motherhood to women (Hays, 1996; Maushart, 1997), the naturalization of women as ideal 'mother workers' (Pande, 2010) requires the treatment of this concept as having always already been the case. Drawing on the work of Marx and Engels, Ahmed makes the point that the distinction between a wooden table (a product) and a tree (a material for production) is arbitrary and a form of strategic naturalization. There is nothing inherent to a tree that predetermines its role as designed for making tables, abstract from a worldview where tables should be made, or where trees should be cut down in the service of humans. Similarly, there is nothing inherent to women that should make them ideally situated to gestate children for others. Rather, this is a product of a strategic naturalization whereby not only is motherhood seen as 'natural', but where women's bodies are seen as natural materials in the service of producing goods (in the case of surrogacy, children for other people).

Our argument here, then, is of a kind with that made by Cooper and Waldby (2014), in their suggestion that

> Biomedical technology can be understood as a practice of controlled decontextualization that is able to provoke unsuspected or as yet unrealized actualizations from its living materials by exposing them to novel environmental conditions. In this respect it is always both an abstract and a material intervention into a spectrum of already available material abstractions.
>
> *(p. 13)*

The difference between our account and that of Cooper and Waldby (2014), however, is that along with decontextualization (i.e. abstracting the wombs of women from their bodies and lives), there is a recontextualization (or strategic naturalization) whereby the decontextualization is treated as natural: as a logical follow-on from what are treated as the natural purposes of women's bodies. Mirroring Cooper and Waldby, however, is our suggestion that this recontextualization is part of a spectrum of 'already available abstractions', and these abstractions are the warp and weft of capitalism which serves capital, not humans per se. Kalindi Vora (2015) summarizes this well when she suggests that:

> Before a human kidney or a given task or type of labor can become seemingly unnecessary in its immediate context and therefore available for outsourcing, it must be the object of specific cultural and material practices that establish it as unnecessary.
>
> *(p. 2)*

As we shall explore in greater detail in Chapters 2 and 3, specific women's bodies and the ends to which women themselves may put them to use are made unnecessary through a series of 'specific cultural and material practices' that produce certain women's bodies as viable producers of goods, and indeed goods in and of themselves. Thus, as Teman (2010) suggests:

> The specific ways in which surrogacy is regulated in California, the United Kingdom, and Israel are shaped not only by politics but also by each culture's key values. The liberal allowance for surrogacy in California extols the core values of individualism, capitalism, and the superiority of technology over nature, all values that have been identified … as central to the American cultural approach to childbirth in general.
>
> *(pp. 10–11)*

Of course, hand in hand with the recontextualization of certain women's bodies as materials and goods of capital comes those who then consume the goods that are produced. Before elaborating this point in further detail, though, it is important for us to reiterate our point that the purpose of capitalism is capital, not humans. We reiterate this point in order to minimize us being misread as repeating the trope that women who act as surrogates are dupes, and people who commission surrogacy arrangements are agentic citizens taking advantage of them. Our point, instead, is that within a capitalist logic, producer, good and consumer are all a product of capitalism, even if the effects upon them and their bodies are differentiated. In other words, and as we shall explore in greater detail later in this chapter, capitalism renders vulnerable all who fall under its remit, even if that vulnerability is differentially distributed.

Without pre-empting our argument about vulnerability, in the remainder of this section we focus on how people who commission surrogacy arrangements mitigate potential vulnerability by emphasizing a logic of intentionality, one that accords to them an agentic role; a point we take up further in Chapters 4 and 7. As a hallmark narrative of capitalism, the agentic subject is one who determines what will matter to them, makes decisions about how to enact what matters to them, and in so doing projects a semblance of a competent self (and see Whittaker, 2015, for a discussion of these issues in relation to reproduction more generally). Given our points earlier about the norm of reproductive citizenship, and specifically the norm of genetic relatedness and the norm of child bearing for women, those who commission surrogacy arrangements are to a certain extent failed reproductive citizens, either due to medical or social infertility. This, at least from our vantage point, indicates how an orientation to surrogacy becomes intelligible for an increasing number of people: the promise of a genetically related child (at least for some intending parents), and a framework through which it is intent (rather than infertility) that leads to the birth of a child. Thus, as Dean Murphy (2015) suggests with regards to the gay couples he interviewed who had entered into surrogacy arrangements: 'In addition to pursuing parenthood according to the marketing of surrogacy agencies, these men are also assuming a particular form of subjectivity: that of responsibilised [*sic*] citizens and reproducers of the population' (p. 121).

Others before us have similarly emphasized how narratives of intent serve to paper over experiences of infertility and assert the agency of intending parents. Vora (2015), for example, suggests that claims to genetic relatedness serve to position 'the commissioning parents as the intentional authors of a future child protected as property, though necessarily under the custodianship of the gestational surrogate for the period of gestation' (p. 40). Key to the work of Ragoné (1994), and indeed framed by the title of her book on the topic of surrogacy, is the idea that surrogacy conception begins 'in the heart, that is, the belief that in the final analysis it [is the intending parents'] desire to have a child that brought the surrogate arrangement into being and therefore produced the child' (p. 126). Heather Jacobson (2016) too emphasizes intent as a mode through which people who have children through surrogacy differentiate themselves from adoptive parents:

> Those in the world of surrogacy resist this adoption framing from the out-set, arguing that because the children were created with the intent of surrogacy, these cases were fundamentally different from adoptive situations. Intent was an important concept from the beginning of third-party reproduction, and it remains so today.
>
> *(p. 18)*

Importantly, however, and in line with the capitalist logic that we argue structures surrogacy, it does not suffice to simply claim intent. Intentionality, like any discourse, is never fixed, and the authors of intent – particularly with regard to surrogacy – can be open to question (consider, for example, the case of Baby M, widely reported in previous literature, which centrally hinged on whose desire brought the child into being). Here, again, the logic of capitalism, which sees the consumer as the agentic subject, plays an important role. Within such a logic, intentionality within surrogacy arrangements is seen as being held primarily if not solely by the intending parents. As Rudrappa (2015) suggests:

> Much as consumers often do not reflect on the labor that goes into making the products they consume in commodity production, the parents too did not ruminate on the surrogate mother's labor. Or if they did, they maintained that she had willingly cut all her ties to the baby upon surrendering it. Engaging in market relations, then, allowed the clients to eliminate the producer. By eliminating her, they recast her labor effort in pregnancy as theirs. And they asserted that they were the baby's true and only parents because this baby existed through their intentions. Through their intentions they had engaged in the market for surrogacy, which had ultimately resulted in this baby.
>
> *(p. 142)*

Further, and as per our suggestion above, not only does the logic of the capitalist market allow intending parents to discount the role of women who act as surrogates as mere producers, but it also allows them to a large extent to discount their own infertility, instead claiming a rightful place within the norm of reproductive citizenship proper. Thus despite claims to the contrary – specifically that surrogacy as an assisted reproductive technology brings into being radically new forms of family (e.g. Appleby & Karnein, 2014) – we follow Strathern (2003) in suggesting that:

> For as long as social ends remain stable, technological innovation does not, in [a] Euro-American (modernist) view have to mean social innovation. On the contrary, as in the promotion of the nuclear family, new procedures may fulfil old goals: the application of technology is taken to have a foundation in social values it leaves unchallenged.
>
> *(p. 292)*

As Strathern emphasizes, surrogacy is an 'assistive' technology. In other words, it does nothing radically new in terms of social norms about the injunction to reproduce, even if the modes of production are somewhat different. Rather, what it does is again naturalize reproduction as an expected part of adulthood, one that allows for entry into adulthood proper, and which is based upon particular roles apportioned to men and women (Riggs & Bartholomaeus, 2017). What slips to the wayside to a certain degree in such an account, and taking up Gayle Rubin's (1975) germinal analysis of the regulation of women and sex, is that the apportioning of specific roles to men and women as 'complementary pairs' functions in the service of capitalism, whereby the couple unit (even if comprised of two men or two women) is tasked with the work of producing children, and thus producing capital. This logic of a natural complementarity is one that we explore in further detail in the next section.

Reproduction and the fantasy of oneness

In some of our other work, and drawing specifically on Lacanian psychoanalysis, we have explored in detail what may be referred to as the fantasy of oneness (Riggs, 2015a). From a Lacanian perspective, before our entrance into language, as infants we perceive ourselves as at one with our primary caregiver. Following the entry, or 'cut', into language, we are fundamentally alienated from this sense of oneness, and it is through our fantasies that we negotiate ways of keeping this feeling of oneness in play. We see this in the idea that searching for a romantic partner constitutes looking for our 'other half', and we also see this in discourses of parenting, particularly in ideas of 'attachment parenting'. To see ourselves as at one with another, at least in fantasy, is to mitigate the sense of alienation that comes from our entry into language.

Given the prevalence of narratives and fantasies such as those described above, it is perhaps unsurprising that they would be evident in discussions about surrogacy. This is most evident in discussions about genetic relatedness, where the bringing together of two gametes, aligned with the intent of the intended parents, produces a one who is the product of two. Of course, we know that at the genetic level this is not accurate: a zygote is formed from *parts* of two gametes, through the process of meiosis. As we have argued elsewhere, 'The zygote that is produced is thus not a "one" produced by two. Instead, it is a one produced by a subtraction from two' (Riggs, 2015a, p. 2). Furthermore, and as twin studies and the study of epigenetics would suggest, there is more at play than simply the combination of two gametes. Multiple factors determine which genes will be activated and in which ways, and this is far more complex than simply one plus one equals one (Gunnarsson Payne, 2016). Further, cases of genetic chimerism – where an individual displays distinctly different chromosomes or blood types within the one body (or in different parts of the body) – suggests that even within ourselves we are not necessarily 'one' (Martin, 2007).

Yet despite the location of claims to oneness in fantasy, and the multiple ways in which they have been disputed by scientific evidence (which of course has no inherent import for our fantasies), they are consistently evoked in the context of surrogacy. A clear example appears repeatedly in cases where one of two intending parents cannot make a genetic contribution to the child being born to them. This may occur within gay cisgender couples, for example, or amongst heterosexual couples where one individual experiences infertility that is not responsive to medical treatment. The work of Murphy (2015) provides multiple examples of the former, where within gay cisgender couples one partner provides the sperm, and the donor eggs are taken from the sister of the other partner, the claim being that the child is thus genetically related to both parents. The assumption in this type of arrangement is that children conceived from two parents share *the same* DNA as their parents, which is a simplified and inaccurate interpretation of genetic inheritance. Whilst they might share *some* DNA inherited from their parents, these are not identical. The work of Thompson (2005) similarly provides examples where heterosexual women, for example, have received donor eggs from their own daughters, the claim being that this then gives them a direct genetic relationship to the child then conceived for them.

In addition to conception being reduced to the simplistic application of Mendelian genetics, intending parents employ other strategies to stake a claim to the idea that 'two becomes one', rather than, for example, three (the intending parents and the woman who acts as the surrogate) or four (the intending parents, the woman who acts as the surrogate, and a gamete donor) differentially make a contribution to 'one'. Teman's (2010) research on surrogacy in Israel provides a key example of this. Teman describes in considerable detail how intending mothers in Israel are treated as though the pregnancy is their own, supplanting any role played by the woman who acts as the surrogate. Similarly, and as we will argue in Chapter 4, some intending parents lay claim to the pregnancy as 'theirs' (i.e. 'we are pregnant', see Riggs & Dempsey, 2015). In multiple and complex ways, then, intended parents lay claim to the pregnancy in ways that, we argue, contribute to the fantasy that 'two become one', reinforcing a sense of oneness within the couple, but also bolstering the claim that the child is solely a product of their intent and/or genetic contribution. As we shall explore in more detail in the following section, it is perhaps understandable, when faced with having 'failed' the norm of reproductivity, that intending parents would seek to position themselves squarely within normative narratives of reproduction. Our concern, however, is with what falls to the wayside in these accounts.

Clearly, the main issue that falls to the wayside in the accounts above is the contribution of women who act as surrogates. As we outlined in the previous section, this falling away is made possible by the logic of capitalism, in which women's bodies can be reduced to mere materials in the service of the production of goods. That intending parents would be co-opted into this narrative is entirely unsurprising. Yet there is more to be made of such co-option. One point of entry into this can be achieved by returning to the processes of meiosis. During the meiosis phase, when two gametes come together, there is a process of combination and stripping, whereby parts of each gamete fall away. This detritus, however, remains as an absent presence. An analogy can be made to cases of 'disappearing twins', where the surviving twin retains traces (sometimes actual body parts) of the absorbed twin within their own bodies. In some of these cases, the absent presence of the lost twin is keenly felt (Riggs & Peel, 2016). What interests us when applying these examples to surrogacy, then, is how women who act as surrogates (and potentially also egg donors) become detritus that fall to the wayside, yet how they nonetheless remain as an absent presence. It is perhaps, we would suggest, anxiety about this absent presence that potentially shapes how intending parents narrate the role of women who act as surrogates and egg donors in the lives of their children. Thus, as Catherine Nash (2015) suggests:

> While the social practice of kinship is performative and flexible, it is worth remembering that kinship is also a classificatory technology that assigns significance to, and orders people within, social groups in terms of degrees of biological connection and distance; that defines categories of inclusion and exclusion; and that differentiates ranks, and naturalizes those exclusions, differentiations, and hierarchies in family and in other collectives.
>
> *(p. 16)*

With regard to surrogacy, the 'performative and flexible' aspects of kinship are vital, given they afford some intending parents ways of, for example, claiming the gestation as their own or laying claim to a genetic contribution to the child. At the same time, however, it would appear that some intending parents rely upon practices of exclusion and differentiation, so as to render only their role and their intent as salient. Ignored in these types of practices is the potential that exists for recognizing multiple contributions to the lives of children. For example, and as Jenny Gunnarsson Payne (2016) suggests with regards to epigenetics and surrogacy:

> If taken further … might even speculate whether, because there is nothing intrinsically bilineal about epigenetics, it might even open up possibilities for thinking through multilineal kinship structures when more than two reproductive parties are involved in creating new life; perhaps, if we were to take the implications of epigenetics in the context of gestational surrogacy and other forms of third-party reproduction seriously, we might learn to apply this new kinship grammar in a way that opens up possibilities for hitherto unknown ways of conceptualizing biological motherhood.
>
> *(p. 503)*

This type of approach, of course, would require a relinquishing of the fantasy of oneness, and as we know, fantasies are not easily relinquished. Yet as we explore in the following section, even if fantasies of oneness are likely to persist, there are ways in which the vulnerabilities faced by many who are party to surrogacy arrangements may at the very least be acknowledged and engaged with, rather than relegated to the margins.

Vulnerability and facing the other

In this final substantive section of the chapter we draw on the work of Judith Butler (2004) and her engagement with the work of Emmanuel Levinas (Levinas & Kearney, 1986) to consider what we might make of the vulnerability that is produced as a result of the injunction to reproductivity. Before doing so, however, it is important for us to first draw together some of the threads of what we have written above with regard to vulnerability. As we have noted, intended parents are likely at some point to have experienced a sense of vulnerability arising from either medical or social infertility. This, we feel, is an important point to make, however, it is a fraught claim, given the broader framework of capitalism that we have argued for, within which whilst we are all rendered objects of capitalism, some of us are marginalized more than others with respect to this objectification. It is difficult – and this is a tension in much of the work on surrogacy to date – to acknowledge the vulnerability potentially faced by intending parents, whilst at the same time not losing sight of who might potentially have the most to lose in surrogacy arrangements (Riggs & Due, 2013).

Certainly, even work that accords a significant degree of agency to women who act as surrogates still acknowledges that most such women, were they to have alternate options, would not choose to act as surrogates. It can, of course, be argued that women who act as surrogates, even if reduced to 'wombs for hire', stand to benefit financially from the transaction. Yet as Rudrappa (2015) has argued, the benefits don't necessarily outweigh the costs, and cannot be abstracted from the broader social contexts in which their bodies become instrumentalized in the service of others. A further cost is elaborated in the work of Ragoné (1994) and Teman (2010), both of whom detail what many women feel they lose when bearing a child for others on contract. Specifically, both suggest that for many women surrogacy is seen as a viable option due to the perceived relationship they will have with the intended parents. For many of Ragoné's participants, there was a significant sense of loss that accompanied the end of the surrogacy relationship, after which many intending parents distanced themselves from the woman who carried their child. Teman (2010) similarly notes that: 'Surrogates often expect that the alliance formed with their intended mother during the pregnancy will represent the beginning of a lasting friendship or kinship bond. For some, these expectations complicated the post-birth period because their couple had contrasting expectations' (p. 206).

Unfortunately for many of Teman's participants, this fear was well-founded. Conducted in the United States and Israel respectively, Ragoné and Teman's work reflects at the very least the *potential* for relationships to be developed and to continue between women who act as surrogates and intending parents. Rudrappa's (2015) research in India, by comparison, illustrates how the surrogacy industry in India all but prevents any contact between intending parents and the women who carry their children. Whilst in our research we have found that this makes India a desirable destination for many intending parents (Riggs, 2015b), Rudrappa's interviewees suggested that the distance between them and the people they were carrying children for was often experienced as marginalizing and indeed distressing. Again, then, our point here (and in this book more widely) is not to minimize the factors that lead some intending parents to distance themselves from women who act as surrogates, nor is it to privilege the vulnerabilities they may face, but rather to consider how surrogacy as a practice differentially produces vulnerabilities for all involved.

The differential effects of vulnerability, we would argue, are written into surrogacy practices from the onset. As Teman (2010), Rudrappa (2015) and others have demonstrated, women who act as surrogates are instructed to focus their concern on the hardship of the people for whom they will carry children. As Ragoné (1994) notes:

> Programs … foster surrogates' empathy for the couple, portraying couples … as composed of individuals who have suffered a great deal of pain, anxiety, disappointment, and unhappiness owing to their infertility. In conveying this message, programs hope to create in their surrogates not only a heightened degree of sensitivity, empathy, and consideration for their couple but a sense of responsibility and mission as well.
>
> (*p. 40*)

This type of missionary zeal is intended to foster a willingness to hand the child over once they are born, and is also presumed to minimize the distress that may be experienced as a result of this handing over. Rudrappa's research, however, contradicts this supposition, suggesting that for many women there is considerable loss associated with the baby they have gestated being quickly taken away, often with them not having even held the baby. In the Indian context at least, not only are women who act as surrogates treated as producers within a context of capitalism, but they are thoroughly alienated from the outcomes of their labour (perhaps because, as we argued earlier, they are not viewed as producers of labour at all, but rather simply as raw materials).

The narrative of missionary zeal is also applied to intending parents, however in different ways. The construction of women who act as surrogates as 'poor' and as in needing of help serves to legitimate the decisions that intending parents make, by minimizing the psychological aspects of gestating a child for another person in favour of discourses which focuses on 'helping' them in relation to money. That many intending parents appear to take up missionary narratives may reflect multiple factors, including the ways in which surrogacy clinics themselves promote these narratives, the ways in which such narratives position intending parents as agentic, and the role that such narratives may play in minimizing any concerns that intending parents may have about the commodification of women who act as surrogates.

How, then, with all of these competing and vexed concerns about caring for others, do we even consider having an orientation to surrogacy that acknowledges multiple forms of vulnerability? Butler's (2004) work on vulnerability and precarity, we believe, offers us a way to think about how, in orienting ourselves to the topic of surrogacy, we must in fact maintain a capacity for multiple orientations. Certainly, as we have signalled in this chapter, our key orientation is to the logic of capitalism. This, however, is a structuring framework. Within that framework it is possible for us to think about what it means to turn towards ourselves as objects of capitalism, whilst at the same time turning towards others who are differentially made objects of capitalism. As we outlined earlier, as parents ourselves, and with regard to our own journeys to and with parenthood, we too are objects of capitalism differentially located with respect to the norm of genetic reproductivity. One of us might in the past have been referred to as a 'surrogate parent', and one of us is frequently subjected to assumptions about what it means to be the 'right kind' of mother. Yet we nonetheless occupy positions of considerable privilege, located outside of the realm of surrogacy in terms of how it is experienced, but certainly not located outside of it in terms of social norms about the 'proper' uses of women's bodies and the operations of capitalism.

Despite our own differing positionings and the differing positionings of the lives of the people whose experiences we explore in this book, Butler (2004) offers us a means through which to develop a conceptual framework that allows for multiple orientations to the vulnerabilities produced by the injunction to reproduction under capitalism. Whilst Butler's work is focused on precarity produced in the context of the 'war on terror', her broader orientation to what it means to locate oneself in a relationship to others lends itself well to the topic of surrogacy. Engaging with the Levinasian conceptualization of the 'face of the Other', Butler (2004) suggests that:

> To respond to the face, to understand its meaning, means to be awake to what is precarious in another life, or rather, the precariousness of life itself. This cannot be an awakeness, to use his word, to my own life, and then an extrapolation from an understanding of my own precariousness to an understanding of another's precarious life. It has to be an understanding of the precariousness of the Other.
>
> *(p. 134)*

This is a complex quote that requires some unpacking. In referring to the 'face' of the Other, Butler is not referring to the actual faces of specific others. Rather, she is referring, following Levinas, to what might be called the 'fact' of the Other, an Other with whom we are always already in a relationship. This is an Other, on par with the psychoanalytic Other, through whom we become intelligible, an Other from whom comes an injunction to recognition in order to ourselves be recognized. Yet as Butler suggests, this recognition cannot start from the place of the self. Rather, we might suggest, recognition must start from an understanding of the fact that without the Other, there is no self. Reaching out to any other actual person, then, whether with love, hatred, an injunction, or a plea, is always already to have acknowledged that the Other as a founding precept makes our reaching out possible. As Butler (2004) goes on to suggest:

> Discourse makes an ethical claim upon us precisely because, prior to speaking, something is spoken to us. In a simple sense, and perhaps not quite as Levinas intended, we are first spoken to, addressed, by an Other, before we assume language for ourselves. And we can conclude further that it is only on the condition that we are addressed that we are able to make use of language. It is in this sense that the Other is a condition of discourse.
>
> *(pp. 138–139)*

The Other that is a 'condition of discourse', then, is both us and not us. It constitutes the very conditions of our entrance into language, but it is also more than just language, more than just any one person. It is the condition by which we speak, and as Levinas argues, the place to which our ethics must be directed. In the case of surrogacy, if the language of the Other is one of precarity (and we would suggest it is, contingent as we all are upon the fantasy of oneness with the Other through which to ground our sense of place in the world), then precarity is the mode by which we address both ourselves and others. Of course, as we suggested above, intending parents may engage in a range of rhetorical strategies aimed at mitigating vulnerability, and surrogacy practices may largely transfer vulnerability onto the shoulders of women who act as surrogates. But this does not mean that the initial mode of address is not precarious. If the face of the Other – and perhaps especially under capitalism – is only intelligible as a face of precarity, then this directs our ethics when it comes to surrogacy. Thus, as Levinas suggests:

> I am defined as a subjectivity, as a singular person, as an 'I', precisely because I am exposed to the other. It is my inescapable and incontrovertible answerability to the other that makes me an individual 'I'. So that I become a responsible or ethical 'I' to the extent that I agree to depose or dethrone myself – to abdicate my position of centrality – in favor of the vulnerable other.
>
> *(Levinas & Kearney, 1986, p. 27)*

Levinas differentiates between the moral and the ethical, suggesting that whilst the former is a set of sociopolitical rules that governs how we interact with one another, the latter emphasizes the fact that our very being is always already oriented towards the Other. To extrapolate to our previous arguments, then, the moral in the context of surrogacy are the sociopolitical rules governed largely by capitalism, in which instrumentalization is made plausible, and where reproductivity is valorized. The ethical, however, is an entirely different matter. It is a matter of 'answerability to the other' that, as Levinas suggests, may require us to challenge the political order 'in the name of our ethical responsibility to the other' (Levinas & Kearney, 1986, p. 30). And this, then, is the orientation that we have argued for, and following Ahmed (2004) again requires a double turn: in turning towards ourselves, we must also turn towards the Other. Both the actual other people upon whose bodies we may rely, but also the face of the Other that produces an imperative for us to be responsible. For to do otherwise – that is, to believe we can turn away from the face of the Other – is to effectively remain stuck as a mere cog in the wheels of capitalism. Such an orientation only serves the purposes of capital, not human life, and means that, in effect, we are turning away from ourselves.

As we shall see in the chapters to come, this understanding of precarity and vulnerability as a foundational aspect of subjectivity provides us with grounds through which to think about the imbrication of all of the groups upon whom we direct our focus. And importantly, whilst those of us not directly involved in surrogacy are not the target of a specific chapter in this book, we are nonetheless implicated in the arguments we make. Our implication as vulnerable subjects faced with the injunction to take up social norms serves to shape our orientation to the topic of surrogacy, and directs our focus towards the aim of acknowledging the role of capitalism, without necessarily treating it as a fait accompli with regard to ways of being in the world and thinking about kinship, connectedness and love.

Chapter overviews

With regard to the content of this book, we first explore in Chapter 2 the conceptual tools that we then apply in the subsequent analytic chapters. Specifically, we map out how human exceptionalism and capitalism combine to produce a context where surrogacy (and the medical technologies that sit behind it) becomes intelligible. In so doing, we consider how certain women's bodies are treated as objects of labour, albeit labour that, due to gender norms, is not quite seen as labour, but rather as a natural predisposition of womanhood. We also explore why medical technologies originally designed to harness the bodies of non-human animals then made the leap to human populations, specifically with regard to, first, the value accorded to having children, and then the value accorded to having genetically related children. We conclude this chapter by outlining how our orientation to the topic of surrogacy fits within a critical health framework, and signal our aim of, in the final analysis, opening up other spaces for thinking about kinship.

Chapter 3 then begins our exploration of various aspects of surrogacy arrangements, by considering data pertaining to women who act as surrogates. Specifically, we explore a documentary featuring the narratives of women living in India who act as surrogates, and advertisements placed on websites by North American women willing to act as surrogates, in order to consider the various orientations to surrogacy displayed by these differing groups of women. Specifically, in this chapter, we discuss the competing discourse seen in these two sources of data concerning women who act as surrogates. In particular, we seek to unpack the competing discourse of 'love or money' in relation to motivations to act as a surrogate, as well as the ways in which women who act as surrogates must represent themselves as desirable to intending parents by portraying themselves as humble, compliant, and often as religious. We conclude by considering how the sociocultural context in which women who act as surrogates live leads to completing claims to what makes a 'good' surrogate, with discourses of helping others, shame and agency often in competition.

In Chapter 4 we turn to consider the orientations that intending parents display towards surrogacy arrangements. In order to do this we consider data from two websites on which intending parents advertise with the aim of meeting women potentially willing to act as surrogates for them, in addition to five self-help books written by people who have had children through surrogacy arrangements. Our analysis of the advertisements suggests that intending parents display complex orientations to the binary of love or money. Specifically, we suggest that intending parents infer that women who act as surrogates should do so out of altruism rather than a desire for money, yet that at the same time the payment of money allows intending parents to 'contract out' of any relationship with the woman carrying their child. From this we suggest that the contracting out of relationships with women who act as surrogates allows intending parents to claim the pregnancy as their own, thus potentially minimizing their reproductive vulnerability.

Having considered both women who act as surrogates and intending parents, in Chapter 5 we examine representations of children born through surrogacy arrangements, and the orientation they are expected to display towards their conception, gestation and birth. We do this through an examination of six storybooks written for children born through surrogacy arrangements. Our analysis suggests that from a young age children born through surrogacy arrangements are directed to view the women who carried them as 'kindly strangers', who 'returned' them to their intending parents. This language of return, following our arguments in Chapter 4, highlights the role of intent in claiming the naturalized rights of intending parents to children born for them in surrogacy arrangements. Also echoing our findings in Chapter 4, our analysis of children's storybooks documents how such books introduce children at an early age to the logic of pronatalism, normalizing the desire for children, and depicting intending parents as first fraught by reproductive vulnerability, only to then overcome this through their agency.

Our focus in Chapter 6 is on surrogacy clinic websites, and specifically the ways in which they market to gay intending parents. Our analysis of twelve such websites suggests that the clinics interpellate gay men into a logic of reproductive citizenship, where genetic relatedness is privileged, and having children is seen as marking the entrance into adulthood proper. The corollary of this, however, is the dual marginalization and instrumentalization of women who act as surrogates, with the websites either making no comment on the role of such women, or treating women as property of the clinic. Our analysis suggests not only that the websites fail to engage with the potential vulnerability of women who act as surrogates, but they also fail to recognize the potential vulnerabilities experienced by intending parents.

Chapter 7 then concludes our analytic chapters through an investigation of representations of surrogacy in public discourse. Specifically, we explore representations of intending parents and the coverage of Baby Gammy within the mainstream Australian media, as well as submissions to a public inquiry concerning surrogacy in New South Wales, Australia. Here, we explore how discourses of vulnerability and intentionality differentially affect intending parents and women who act as surrogates, such that – and as argued above – women who act as surrogates are represented as vulnerable, while intending parents are represented as agentic. In addition, we explore how public representations of surrogacy draw upon normative accounts of women to argue either for or against surrogacy arrangements.

Finally, in Chapter 8 we provide an overview of the findings in our analysis chapters before engaging with the work of various theorists and frameworks to consider ways forward in relation to surrogacy. Importantly, this chapter does not advocate – or even engage with – debates concerning state responsibility in relation to surrogacy legislation or individual attitudes. Instead, we argue for ways in which we can 'open up' marginalized discourses in order to disorient surrogacy itself as a seemingly normalized form of reproduction (both in terms of the creation of children, and in terms of the reproduction of a capitalist logic). In doing so, we aim to explore the ways in which a critical health perspective on surrogacy – as elaborated throughout this book – can create opportunities to promote health equity and well-being for all groups of people engaged in surrogacy arrangements, including a possible orientation *away* from surrogacy.

2

CONCEPTUAL TOOLS

In Chapter 1 we outlined in detail the orientation that we take to the topic of surrogacy, framing our orientation specifically with reference to capitalism as a structuring logic, and vulnerability as a way of thinking through how differing parties are inculcated within this logic. In presenting our orientation, however, we necessarily glossed over some of the broader histories that shape and are shaped by capitalism, and through which surrogacy becomes a mode of having children that is culturally endorsed in neoliberal contexts. In this chapter, then, we explore in greater detail four specific conceptual tools that we believe offer additional analytic leverage for understanding the role of capitalism in shaping an orientation towards surrogacy as an intelligible way of thinking about both women's bodies and having children, and the differential vulnerabilities that this produces. Specifically, we focus on:

1 the intersections of human exceptionalism and pronatalism in the context of reproductive technologies;
2 the ways in which reproductive labour is taken as a naturalized form of gendered work;
3 contemporary narratives of children as priceless, and the historical antecedents to this; and
4 the value attached to genetic relatedness.

We conclude the chapter by connecting all four of these conceptual tools to the understanding of wellbeing that we utilize in subsequent chapters, specifically by connecting 'health' not to individual bodies, but rather to the structuring logics by which certain ways of being are rendered intelligible as forms of 'living well'.

Human exceptionalism

In our previous work on critical kinship studies (Riggs & Peel, 2016), we have argued that understanding human kinship practices requires an understanding of the role of human exceptionalism (i.e. the assumption that humans are the most important beings living on the planet, and that it is therefore reasonable that our ways of being are treated as the most valued). Specifically, we have suggested that thinking about how and why humans reproduce cannot be abstracted from the value accorded to human life (and as we shall argue below, specific human lives) at the expense of the lives of other species, and indeed the planet itself. Starting from, for example, how some humans decide to have children, or how surrogacy has become an intelligible mode of family formation, is thus to start halfway through the story. Ultimately, we suggest, the story of human reproduction starts a long way before the decisions that actual humans make as to whether or not and how we have children. Instead, we suggest, and following the work of those who have mapped some of the historical intersections between human and non-human reproduction outlined below, it is vital to understand the legacies upon which contemporary reproductive practices rest.

Given the intersections in the histories that we briefly map in this section, it is difficult to discern which comes first: the instrumentalization of non-human animals, or the instrumentalization of particular humans. For our purposes, we will start with the former and work our way through to arguments about the latter. Specifically, we first draw upon the work of Sarah Franklin (2001) and Melinda Cooper (2008), both of whom have focused extensively on how reproductive science as applied to non-human animals has centrally informed the development of reproductive technologies as used on humans, though as Franklin suggests, the relationship between the two is circular, with a constant back and forth between the two fields.

Cooper (2008), drawing on the work of Adele Clarke (1998), argues that the development of reproductive technologies as applied to non-human animals has historically been driven by a capitalist logic, namely to increase the controllability of both reproduction and thus the production of goods (such as flesh, milk and eggs). Traditional methods of farming and raising livestock, reliant upon breeding seasons and their relative unreliability, became increasingly unsuitable for meeting the needs of a growing population, in addition to being unsuitable to ensuring a steady, if not increasing, accumulation of capital arising from the capacity to produce and provide goods. Reproductive technologies, then, as they were first applied through experimentation on animals, allowed for the regulation of heritability, first through the identification of ideal sperm that could be harvested and used to inseminate multiple animals (thus ensuring some stability in breed outcomes), and then in the regulation of breeding cycles themselves. Controlling the means of production necessitated controlling the means of reproduction.

In her work with Catherine Waldby, Cooper (2014) has further argued that the regulation of breeding cycles in non-human animals raised for human purposes (i.e. for their reproductive-related products – milk or eggs – or for their very lives in the form of flesh) represents Marxian temporal abstraction par excellence. As Cooper and Waldby note, temporal abstraction enables exchangeable labour, whereby any body can stand in for another in a capitalist logic under which production is most highly valued when it is uniform and guaranteed. Franklin (2001) makes a similar point in her reading of the technologies that made possible the cloning of Dolly the sheep. Through the culturing of what are seen as 'neutral' cells, the idealized material (and, we could argue by extension, the idealized worker) is one that is entirely substitutable, bearing no trace of its own presence, but rather being entirely assimilable into the presence of another (i.e. the consumer).

Yet as Cooper and Waldby (2014) also suggest, all of this work of breaking down the bodies of non-human animals into their component (reproductive) parts so as to facilitate their more ready re-production would be of little value in the absence of a desire or need for the goods that are produced. Hand in hand with the need for animal products, then, has come the creation of a marketplace wherein animal products are desirable (Calvo, 2008). Whilst it is beyond our remit to substantively address this point here, we would note, for example, how the practice of providing milk to school children as part of lunches was historically part of a concerted effort to bolster the agricultural economy in countries such as the United Kingdom (Atkins, 2005). Given the prominent role that agriculture (and animal farming in particular) played in many countries in the early twentieth century, national economies often hinged on the successful uptake of the goods produced as a result of agriculture. Following slumps in sales of milk during the First and Second World Wars, promoting dairy milk as central to a healthy diet, and providing it to school children, was one way of inculcating future consumers into supporting the dairy industry, and into viewing non-human animals as solely existing to service the needs of humans (Cole & Stewart, 2014).

Hand in hand with the instrumentalization of non-human animals and the promotion of the consumption of animals, is the treatment of some humans as less than human, indeed as animals. Central to scientific racism and eugenics was the legitimization of the treatment of certain groups of humans as valuable only for the work to which they could be put (Richards, 2003). Chattel slavery as enacted upon the bodies and lives of people trafficked from the African continent foreshadowed and was complicit with some of the logics that were later applied in the development of reproductive sciences as applied to non-human animals. Not only were humans purchased as slaves valued only for the work they could produce, but forced reproduction was used as a means to increase the numbers of people that were owned by any individual. Following the end of the slave trade in the eighteenth century, forced reproduction (including through rape by owners) was a key means through which slave holdings could be increased (Bridgewater, 2001).

As we suggested above, then, reproductive technologies as applied to non-human animals serve the purposes of human exceptionalism. Further, as we noted above, the 'human' in human exceptionalism has historically, and indeed still in the present, been only applied to a limited group of humans. Whilst pronatalism, as we explore in more detail in the following section, is a key outcome of human exceptionalism (i.e. the axiomatic idea that as humans we should reproduce ourselves), whose reproductivity is valued is highly contingent upon which human lives are valued. Whereas the reproductivity of enslaved humans, for example, was valued solely as it allowed owners to increase their workforce (and thus increase their capital through increased output), such reproductivity in turn made possible the privileged role accorded to reproduction by those who were not slaves (i.e. white people).

Without wishing to pre-empt the sections that follow, we can close this section by noting that human exceptionalism is reliant upon the instrumentalization not only of non-human animals, but also of certain humans who are considered or positioned as somehow less than human. As we noted above, however, this does not mean that the reproductivity of those considered less than human is not valued. Rather, their reproductivity is a cornerstone of the capitalist market in which the bodies of some humans become materials in the production of goods to be consumed by others. In our examples above we referred specifically to chattel slavery, and without wishing to minimize the totalistic ways in which slavery denied the embodied personhood of those humans treated as slaves, there are certainly other examples where the reproductivity of some is valued solely for the purposes of others. Clearly, as is the focus of the book, surrogacy is such an example. As with the history of reproduction in the agricultural sciences, leading to developments in technologies applied to human reproduction, surrogacy builds upon the technologies that preceded it.

A further example of the technologies that preceded surrogacy as currently practised, again following Cooper and Waldby (2014), is human gametes and their increasing disaggregation from human bodies, whereby abstraction allows for the production of capital. Although Cooper and Waldby argue that, despite the similarities between developments in agricultural reproduction and human reproduction, there is still something of a fundamental difference between the two in terms of the extent of commodification, we would more concertedly argue that commodification functions very similarly across the two markets. As we have argued above, both markets (i.e. agricultural reproduction and human reproductive technologies) work in the service of human exceptionalism, which more broadly serves the purposes of capitalism. As Cooper and Waldby (2014) themselves note with regard to sperm donation, donor programmes promote an understanding of 'human genetic capital', allowing each donor to see themselves as bringing 'a portfolio of desirable entrepreneurial, intellectual, physical, and psychological attainments to the task of gamete production' (p. 43). On the one hand, then, sperm donors are entrepreneurs, marketing themselves through the promotion of desirable characteristics (many of which, Cooper and Waldby argue, are not actually genetically determined, but which are instead accorded a patina of genetic importance). On the other hand, their reproductive capacity is deemed meritorious within a capitalist logic whereby individual embodied materials can be abstracted and sold on the market. As we shall see in the following section, such processes of abstraction are specifically gendered with regard to women's roles in practices of surrogacy.

Gendered work

In the previous section we focused on human exceptionalism, largely taking the category 'human' as an homogenous entity. In this section, however, we further problematize this category, specifically with regard to gender. Given the fundamental (though not inherently correct) association of sperm with men and ovum with women, it is nothing new to note that reproductivity is gendered (Martin, 1991). Nor, as we do in this section, is it anything new to note that cisgender women bear the greatest weight of the injunction to reproductivity. Nonetheless, what we seek to do in this section is to map out some of the competing (though not inherently contradictory) discourses that function to position certain women's bodies as more prone than others to commodification. We argue that this commodification results, not because of something inherent about their bodies per se (though certainly, that argument is often made), but rather because of how their bodies are positioned within capitalism more broadly. Moreover, we seek to explore why it is that certain women's bodies are rendered intelligible objects of surrogacy, given the following point made so eloquently by Leta Hollingworth as early as 1916:

> The facts, shorn of sentiment, then, are: (1) The bearing and rearing of children is necessary for tribal or national existence and, aggrandizement. (2) The bearing and rearing of children is painful, dangerous to life, and involves long years of exacting labor and self-sacrifice. (3) There is no verifiable evidence to show that a maternal instinct exists in women of such all-consuming strength and fervor as to impel them voluntarily to seek the pain, danger, and exacting labor involved in maintaining a high birth rate.
>
> *(pp. 20–21)*

How, then, and given the likely costs to themselves, are women compelled to take up the injunctions of pronatalism? Betty Rollin (1974) provides a potted history of how it is that the role of women in reproduction is naturalized:

> Originally, it was the word of God that got the ball rolling with 'Be fruitful and multiply', a practical suggestion, since the only people around then were Adam and Eve. But in no time, super-moralists like St. Augustine changed the tone of the message … So then and now, procreation took on a curious value among people who viewed the pleasures of sex as sinful. One could partake in sinful pleasure, but feel vindicated by the ensuing birth. Motherhood cleaned up sex. Also, it cleaned up women, who have always been considered somewhat evil … And so, based on need, inevitability and pragmatic fantasy, the Myth [of motherhood] worked. In fact, the Myth persisted, breaking some kind of record for long-lasting fallacies.
>
> *(pp. 149–150)*

Rollins' somewhat tongue-in-cheek account provides us with the contours of what we flesh out in this section, namely how it is that motherhood and womanhood are collapsed into one, and yet how surrogacy (in which a woman bears a child and then hands them over to another person) is rendered intelligible within a framework of womanhood that would otherwise see women who act as surrogates as discredited women. Certainly, we are not claiming that such discrediting does not happen, given that across the literature there are many examples of women who act as surrogates reporting being positioned as failed women (see Markens, 2007; Roach Anleu, 1992, for an overview). Rather, our point in this section is to explore how, despite norms of motherhood and negative constructions of women who act as surrogates, so many women agree to act as surrogates, and how this becomes naturalized. Specifically, in this section we focus on how a binary appears to operate, whereby certain women are positioned as those required to take up the injunction to pronatalism, whilst other women are positioned as service providers whose role it is to prop up the infertility of women who are normatively expected to reproduce. It is this binary, we suggest, that appears to allow for flexibility in what is otherwise the rigidly defined expectation that women who bear children also mother children. Similar to our point in the previous section, then, human exceptionalism is founded upon the assumption that certain humans count more than others, and certain humans are more open to incorporation as goods under capitalism rather than as consumers (see also Whittaker & Speier, 2010).

A key example of how certain women are positioned as goods under capitalism appears in the research of Rudrappa (2015), who outlines extensively how programmes for the sterilization of women (via tubal ligation) in India have served to produce a population of women who are now seen as viable objects by surrogacy agencies. The practice of sterilization, Rudrappa suggests, is produced within histories where Indian women's bodies are devalued, and leads to contemporary practices whereby, due to experience and skills in population control programmes, Indian doctors are highly experienced in working upon women's bodies. Importantly, Rudrappa suggests that programmes of sterilization implemented amongst poor, rural communities in India from the 1960s onwards were often bolstered via funding received from the United States. Here, then, we have histories wherein the United States funded the very circumstances that now render certain Indian women's bodies intelligible as sources of labour for (often American) people experiencing infertility.

The sterilization of Indian women who subsequently act as surrogates for women from other countries provides an interesting counter to narratives about what leads women from other countries to enter into surrogacy arrangements. For some such women (and for cisgender gay men), infertility may be what leads them to surrogacy arrangements. Yet for some women, surrogacy arrangements may follow decisions to delay creating a family until after establishing a career, by which point the woman's reproductive capacity may have decreased. Importantly, our suggestion here is not that all women should want to have children, nor that they should do so at a younger age. We are very mindful that gender imbalances in the labour force mean that women must increasingly work harder than their male counterparts to achieve outcomes that are still often not on a par with those of men. Nonetheless, it is notable to us that whilst certain groups of Indian women have children at a younger age before going into service industries where they act as surrogates, women from other countries may do the opposite, and there is a seemingly inverse relationship between the cultural capital held by each group of women.

Furthermore, and to return to the points we made in the previous section about slavery and forced reproduction, we might wish to compare and contrast the rights of certain women to have children and for this to be supported by the state (in the case of middle-class, often white, women), and the rights of women not to undergo involuntary (or coerced) sterilization. As Dorothy Roberts (2002) notes, there is a tension underpinning the right to choose (in regard to abortion, for example): namely, that whilst certain (white) women are compelled not to abort children under the name of either pronatalism or religious convictions, other (for example, Indian or African American) women are compelled not to *have* children, or to risk their children being removed from their care due to culturally biased perceptions of abuse or neglect. As these examples suggest, then, the generic 'womanhood equals motherhood' narrative is perhaps not as generic as it may seem. Rather, it is a narrative that is specifically applied to certain women, and when other women take up the narrative, their experiences are problematized.

Yet whilst the apportioning of reproductive labour to certain women in the service of other people may indeed be seen as a form of material production under capitalism, research consistently suggests that women who act as surrogates experience an injunction not to perceive their labour as work. As Heather Jacobson (2016) suggests:

> Selecting women who display a proper orientation to surrogacy – one not focused on money, but on altruistic giving and a love of pregnancy – is an important strategy employed by surrogacy agencies and those lawyers and reproductive endocrinologists who broker matches between [intending parents] and surrogates. For surrogacy to function properly, money cannot be the explicitly stated primary goal, I was told over and over again in my interviews with agency owners and workers, surrogates, and their family members.
>
> *(p. 160)*

Arguably missing from Jacobson's account, however, is the word 'gendered': 'a proper[ly gendered] orientation to surrogacy'. What Jacobson appears to be referring to are broader cultural norms about womanhood, in which women bear and birth children not for money, but for love. This is what we suggest is a properly gendered orientation to surrogacy, one that enshrines a normative account of womanhood, whilst at the same time implicitly constructing what becomes defined as the ideal 'mother worker' (Pande, 2010): a woman who bears a child 'like a woman' (i.e. for love, not for money), but who accepts that commerce frames the pregnancy and birth.

Yet as Roach Anleu (1992) suggests, this ability to conform to norms of womanhood whilst also accepting a capitalist framing of reproductive labour is not an especially novel set of expectations placed upon women. Given women are normatively expected to care and give to others, then caring and giving, even if they come with financial compensation, are not entirely foreign to normative accounts of womanhood (Zelizer, 2005). What would be atypical, however, would be a woman who privileges the financial transaction over the purported caring and loving aspects of a pregnancy, or indeed who discounts the latter entirely. However, both Ragoné (1994) and Jacobson (2016) suggest that women who focus primarily on surrogacy as a means to making money are vetted during initial interviews with surrogacy agencies, with those deemed to have what is constituted as an inappropriate orientation to surrogacy excluded. We explore these tensions between love and money further in the next chapter.

What we have argued in this section, then, is that there are a number of historical and contemporary antecedents that position certain women's bodies as those most appropriate for the practice of surrogacy. Whilst these are bodies that are typically financially compromised, however, the transactional aspects of the surrogacy arrangement are expected to be minimized, in favour of a narrative that emphasizes the normatively expected maternal feelings of care and altruism. As such, accounts of surrogacy typically minimize any understanding of surrogacy as a form of transactional labour, whilst at the same time being reliant upon the fact that certain women's bodies are more vulnerable to commerce than others. This is achieved through the naturalization of women's reproductive capacities within many cultures, rather than as a capacity that is enhanced and enacted through cultural practices that emphasize normatively expected roles for men and women. Whilst we have referred to this as 'gendered work', then, the 'work' apportioned to women in the context of surrogacy is that which is normatively expected of them, and hence can be dismissed as not truly being work (even if, as Murphy, 2015, suggests in his research, that some intending parents do indeed dismiss the labour of surrogacy as simply paid work). Arguably what is at stake in these competing framings, and as we explore in more detail in the following section, is the outcome of surrogacy arrangements, namely children. How we value children and the circumstances it is acceptable through which to have children (i.e. love, not money), provides us with a further understanding of how surrogacy is framed less as 'work' (as the word is normatively understood), and more as something certain women can, and indeed should, do.

Priceless children

Thus far we have argued that an orientation towards surrogacy as a way of having children is shaped by a capitalist logic that differentially renders people vulnerable to the pronatalist injunction to reproduce. Yet missing from this equation is an important question: why do people want to have children in the first place? Certainly in our research on heterosexual couples planning for a first child (Riggs &

Bartholomaeus, 2016) we have found that such couples typically make recourse to claims about having children as 'natural' and 'innate', but what exactly do these words mean? Moreover, and as we address in this section, how have children become so sought after, to such an extent that for many people they have become the holy grail of adulthood proper?

Children have not always been viewed in the ways they are today. In his classic text *Centuries of Childhood*, Phillipe Ariès (1962) maps out something of the trajectory of the construction of childhood, and by extension children, as a valued category. As is the case with many topics, Ariès suggests a degree to which contemporary understandings of children are reworkings of those which have come before. So, for example, Ariès draws a distinction between the 'coddled' child and the morally managed child. The former, he suggests, was most salient in the sixteenth century where, at least in families who could afford to, children were treated as cherished objects, lavished with considerable attention from their parents, and especially their mothers. Throughout the seventeenth century, however, and continuing through into the eighteenth century, religious moralists increasingly sought to regulate the degree of affection shown towards children by their parents, instead emphasizing children as born with natural sin that required taming.

Importantly, however, and as we hinted at above, many of the narratives of childhood that Ariès explores (1962) are slanted towards the practices of families with the necessary financial means to see children either as objects to coddle, or objects to tame. Other, and particularly poor, families, had (and continue to have) far fewer choices in terms of the options available for determining and enacting particularly pathways for their children. Yet despite these differences arising from financial resources, Zelizer (1994) suggests that throughout the nineteenth century and most certainly in the early decades of the twentieth century there was a degree to which the ways in which children were viewed across differing families converged upon an idea of children as objects to be managed. In saying this, of course, we do not wish to minimize the vast differences between the lives of children in differing social groups. The lives of children working in mines, for example, were vastly different to the lives of children expected to attend school and enter into family businesses. What unites these experiences, however, is an increased focus on the role of children in the labour market, either as income earners in their own right, or as future income earners. It is through this shift in viewing children as resources and thus either as assets or as liabilities that we can see the increasing role of capitalism shaping the lives of parents and children.

Of course, as we noted in the previous section, and particularly with regard to the injunction to reproduce, there is the vexed issue of who historically (and still in the present) were positioned as desirable parents, and who were not. Combined with this, however, was now the issue of who were desirable children (i.e. those who were an asset) and who were not. Given the lack of effective birth control methods at the turn of the nineteenth century, the rapid growth of populations in Western countries, and the lack of social security for most families, the stage was set for children to become a considerable concern in terms of the inability or unwillingness of certain families, as well as the state, to care for them. In her work on this era, Zelizer (1994) carefully documents how the state was presented with a significant problem in terms of the high numbers of children who were abandoned by their parents (because they simply could not afford to raise them), and the relatively limited number of families who were willing to take such children in. Whilst older children could be taken in as servants, infants and younger children were wholly seen as a liability, rather than as a potential future asset. As Zelizer discusses, this led to the practice of 'baby farming', where parents could surrender their children for a fee to someone who would notionally raise them, yet many of the children 'sold' in this way were left to die, or were cruelly mistreated.

Faced with the growing numbers of children who were abandoned, and public outcry over baby farming, Zelizer (1994) suggests that in the United States governments were faced with the dilemma of how to make children desirable to parents once again. One response was to introduce social security payments for mothers, though this was considered by many to potentially exacerbate the issue rather than solve it. Another response, and one that is key to the trajectory we are mapping out here, was to attempt to shift public perceptions away from seeing children as a liability or abandoned children as only viable to care for if they could be an asset in terms of the labour they produced. Instead, welfare agencies and church groups emphasized what were depicted as the inherent benefits to raising children. Whilst this was of a kind with Ariès' (1962) notion of the coddled child, it was different in that this was a state-sanctioned narrative about the value of children, and the importance of seeing children not as chattels, but rather as precious love objects.

This type of narrative about children not only promoted the idea that having children was a laudable aim, but also promoted the idea that raising children born to another person (i.e. through adoption) was a socially acceptable means through which to become a parent. Obviously this narrative was not uniformly true, and certainly as we will explore in the following section there was and continues to be a hierarchy through which certain modes of having children are more valued than others. Nonetheless, promoting the inherent value of children served to address concerns about baby farming, and to turn the tide away from the view that children were potential liabilities, to the view that children were assets in their own rights (i.e. as objects of love and of status). Aiding this understanding of children as love objects was the rise of behaviourism in the early decades of the twentieth century, which emphasized, in effect, nurture over nature, positing that we are all the products of external stimuli. This logic was important to the state agenda of increasing the number of people willing to raise children not born to them: if adoptive parents could shape and mould the behaviours of children placed with them, then they too could form loving families that largely mirrored those formed through reproductive heterosex.

It would of course be remiss of us if we did not comment on some of the other apparatus that then sat around the idea of children as precious and priceless. Viewing children in this way reinforced at least two factors that were already evident in capitalist societies at the time. First, the role of mothers was further enshrined as central to the wellbeing of children, with the work of mothering naturalized as something that women automatically do, which served to justify the continued exclusion of women from the workforce. Whilst, as the decades of the twentieth century progressed, and certainly following the Second World War, women increasingly entered the workforce, it would be fair to say that women have continued to face an injunction to raise children, and judgements about women who are not mothers, or who are mothers but who work full-time, continue to be wielded against such women (Maushart, 1997). A focus on children as precious and priceless, then, has served to add legitimacy to what are seen as natural differences between men and women, and thus to justify the apportioning of the majority of care work to women.

The second factor reinforced through the idea of children as precious and priceless is the growth of consumerism. Along with a focus on children as precious and priceless has come an understanding that 'good parents' and 'happy children' require the endless plethora of items marketed to them. In this sense, then, there was a shift from seeing children as solely producers of labour, to seeing children as warranting consumption, and indeed children as consumers themselves (Langer, 2002). Here, then, we can see the outlines of a logic wherein children have become increasingly enmeshed with the operations of capitalism and consumption, and thus it is no great stretch to understand why it is the case not only that children are desirable, but that a market in surrogacy services has become viable. In other words, the logic of consumption no longer begins after a child is born, rather it is a logic that, in the case of surrogacy perhaps most clearly, drives the desire to have children in the first place. Yet as we will explore further in the following section, it is not simply a drive to have children as part of a broader logic of consumerism. Rather, it is a drive to have a particular kind of child: one to whom one is genetically related.

Genetic relatedness

Hand in hand with the state-endorsed narrative of children being precious and priceless (albeit, as we will explore further below, focused on a particular – middle-class – segment of society) has come the proliferation of groups of people seeking to have children, groups who historically were excluded from having children. Whilst historically infertile heterosexual couples were able to adopt, and more latterly to access assisted reproductive technologies, it is only very recently that other groups – and specifically lesbians and gay men – have had access to either adoption or reproductive technologies. On the one hand, the increased access to assisted reproductive technologies by a broader range of groups with regard to having children has been celebrated by these groups, whilst on the other hand, the diversification of family forms has led to a bolstering of arguments (such as by the Christian right) against increased access. In this section we focus on how an emphasis on genetic relatedness, as it has grown exponentially in the latter decades of the twentieth century, has served the purposes of naturalizing a particular form of kinship, with surrogacy providing a key example of this.

In their study of what they refer to as the 'DNA mystique', Dorothy Nelkin and M. Susan Lindee (2004) suggest that:

> Increasing popular acceptance of genetic explanations and the proliferation of genetic images reflects, in part, highly publicized research in the science of genetics. Such research, however, occurs in a specific cultural context, one in which heredity and natural ability have often seemed important to formulations of social policy and social practice. Old ideas have been given new life at a time when individual identity, family connections, and social cohesion seem threatened and the social contract appears in disarray.
>
> *(p. 3)*

As they suggest, the rise of genetic science – what Kaja Finkler (2000) refers to as the 'hegemony of the gene' (p. 3) – came at a time not simply when technologies had developed to the point where this was possible, but at a time when social norms and conventions were in flux. The search for the truth of the question of kinship in the forms of genetics, then, was a solution to the problem as to what best to affix 'old ideas' to, namely to once again affirm existing social contracts through linking them to genetics. The supposed naturalness of reproductive heterosex, the supposed automatic union of sperm and egg, and the supposed natural roles of men and women could all be affirmed through genetic science. This was possible, as Nelkin and Lindee suggest, because:

> The notion of the molecular family is based on the cultural expectation that a biological entity can determine emotional connections and social bonds – that can link us to each other and somehow preserve a reliable model for a family. Since it is beyond culture, outside of DNA seems to be of durable or permanent significance. Genetic ties seem to ground family relationships in a stable and well defined unit, providing the individual with indisputable roots more reliable than the ephemeral ties of love, friendship, marital vows, or shared values.
>
> *(2004, p. 60)*

Certainly, as many have since argued (e.g. Franklin, 2013; Nash, 2015), genetics are as much a product of a specific cultural moment as are any other claims that are naturalized as being prior to culture. Yet this has not stopped genetic science becoming the new natural, referring here specifically to the way in which cultural constructs become grounded in claims that are seen as absolute truths about the world around us. One implication of this, and as Nelkin and Lindee explore, has been the discounting of kinship forms that do not involve genetic relatedness. Specifically, Nelkin and Lindee suggest that with the rise of genetic determinism has come the further marginalization of, for example, adoption or fostering. Thus, whilst in the previous section we suggested that the narrative of children as precious and priceless opened the door for adoption as a means to combat baby farming, in this section we suggest that adoption as a legitimate mode of family formation has, at least to a degree, been supplanted by the proliferation of ways to have children in which at least one of the parents are genetically related to the child, or where a patina of genetic relatedness can be claimed (see also Ginsburg & Rapp, 1991; Finkler, 2000).

As Nelkin and Lindee (2004) suggest, surrogacy provides an answer to concerns about adoption as not engendering a 'real' connection between parents and children (when 'real' is defined by genetic relatedness), and also provides women (and indeed in some cases men) with the vicarious experience of pregnancy, which too has become increasingly lauded as essential to the experience of becoming a parent (as we explore in more detail in Chapter 4). Whilst historically pregnancy was seen as a risk to women, and as a necessary evil as part of having children, today pregnancy is lauded as an idealized part of becoming parents for those who cannot bear children themselves (Teman, 2010). Of course, in the case of surrogacy, pregnancies are undertaken by people other than the intending parents. Thus, whilst pregnancy might be idealized and experienced vicariously by intending parents, this does not change that pregnancies can still be a risk for women. Further, it does not mitigate that women who act as surrogates are made vulnerable to this risk precisely in the service of other people gaining a genetically related child and the desire to vicariously experience pregnancy.

To return to our focus in Chapter 1 on orientations to surrogacy, Jacobson (2016) suggests that the development of reproductive technologies, and especially in vitro fertilization (IVF) specifically applied to gestational surrogacy, have served to warrant an orientation to surrogacy framed as fulfilling the idealized norm of genetically related families:

> The contemporary surrogacy industry walks a fine line between expanding and increasing its profitability, on the one hand, and remaining culturally palatable by fitting into cultural norms about family reproduction, on the other hand. The development of IVF was crucial for balancing these twin market demands, for it is not only a highly profitable medical procedure, creating a huge market and attracting new industry players, but it also allows for a reiteration of genetic kinship ties that fits nicely with normative ideologies of the family in the United States. Traditional surrogacy, in which the surrogate used her own egg, challenged these basic normative ideas popular in the United States that equate true parenthood with genetic lineage. With IVF, that challenge is eliminated as both intended fathers and intended mothers are able to enact genetic parenthood.
>
> *(p. 42)*

The ability for intended parents, at least in some cases, to 'enact genetic parenthood' has led to some such parents believing that surrogacy positions them at the leading edge of contemporary kinship forms, through their evocation of agency, intentionality and genetics, as Rudrappa (2015) suggests: 'Many intended parents I interviewed – straight or otherwise – believe they are moral pioneers because they are progenitors of a new kind of mestizo/a, encompassing vastly divergent genetic genealogies' (p. 7).

Certainly, and following the work of Thompson (2005), Rudrappa is correct in suggesting that the ways in which intending parents combine genetic narratives to their own ends positions them as akin to pioneers. Gay cisgender couples who use ovum from one of the men's sisters, for example, or heterosexual cisgender women who use their daughter's ovum, find increasingly novel ways to lay claim to genetic relatedness. Yet we would also insist that in their broadest sense none of these strategies are particularly new with regard to the logic that underpins them. If children are seen as precious and priceless, then the desire to have children and to promote this as the pinnacle of one's life is nothing new, even in the context of surrogacy arrangements. Furthermore, given the fact that genetic relatedness is not a reflection of an external truth, but rather a very particular cultural construction of kinship (Schneider, 1968), then it is unsurprising that those who enter into surrogacy arrangements will find new ways of repeating this same truth claim.

As Finkler (2000) suggests, genetics become a proxy for the somewhat unusual pairing of destiny and intent. Specifically, genetic relatedness allows for the mapping of traits across generations so that their expression in any given individual becomes a matter of genetic destiny (see Nash, 2015), whilst the intentional enactment of genetic relatedness (such as in the context of surrogacy) gives destiny a purposive flavour, a hallmark of neoliberal citizenship where one can be both destined to take a particular life pathway (i.e. have a child), yet at the same time make agentic decisions about how to achieve this. Whilst claims to destiny are also made in the context of other modes of family formation (such as foster care, see Riggs, Delfabbro & Augoustinos, 2009), the hegemony of the gene provides a contemporary and privileged way of accounting for destiny.

There is, of course, another side to the story of those who enter into surrogacy arrangements as intending parents, and who may see themselves as 'moral pioneers' (Rudrappa, 2015, p. 7). The side of the story that is often marginalized is the labour of those who contribute to such alleged pioneering. Obviously in this book we are focused primarily on women who act as surrogates, and this point about marginalization is one that we have already stated clearly with regard to women who act as surrogates (and will explore further in Chapter 3). A further point, however, must be made with regard to women who donate their ovum for the purposes of surrogacy arrangements. As Jacobson (2016) notes above, 'traditional' surrogacy was problematic because the woman who carried the child also had a genetic relationship to the child. This led to cases (such as that of Baby M), where the woman then claimed a parental relationship to the child after they were born. The genetics of others, then, was a problem. The advent of ovum donation and the ability to create embryos in vitro, it is often believed, addressed this issue, by separating out creation from gestation. Yet this type of belief belies the fact that when donor ovum are used (as is almost always the case for gay men, and is increasingly the case for heterosexual couples where the female partner does not have viable ovum), the genetics of the donor form part of the story.

To manage the threat that donor gametes potentially present to the destined intent of people who have children through surrogacy arrangements, Lauren Jade Martin (2015) argues that intending parents often make recourse to selective claims about genetic determinism when framing their accounts of donor selection. Donor ovum are often taken as a synecdoche for the entire woman, who is then taken as a representative of a particular social grouping, whether that be in regards to religion, ethnicity or class. As she suggests:

> The genetic imperative is not always about passing on one's own genetic material. Sometimes it is about passing on the genetic material of one who is racially, ethnically, or phenotypically similar ... If one can't pass on one's own genetic material, the next best thing is, perhaps, to have some control over whose genes will be passed on.
>
> *(Martin, 2005, p. 142)*

The process of selecting donor eggs, much like the process of selecting donor sperm, as Laura Mamo (2007) found in her research, brings with it complex determinations about how to best approximate genetic relatedness (Kroløkke, 2014). Specifically, such determinations follow a pathway through which the donor stands in for a group of which the recipient is a member, who can then lay claim to the genes themselves. Yet these determinations are complex, we would suggest, following Murphy (2015), precisely because, having first established the importance of genetics in determining relatedness, intending parents who use donated gametes must then go on to discount the role of the donor. Certainly this does not necessarily occur in every case of surrogacy, but replete across the literature are examples of a paired contrast between the importance of genetic relatedness in terms of the intentions of the intending parents, and a discounting of the genetic contribution made by the egg donor (and to a certain extent the biological contribution of the woman who acts as a surrogate). As we argued above, whilst there is a particular logic through which claims are made to the genetic material of another as one's own – and certainly the logic of genetic inheritance as Nash (2015) so clearly maps out allows for these types of claims – the logic nonetheless brings with it the spectre of *failing* to truly occupy a place within the norm of genetic relatedness.

Whilst the spectre of failing is potentially omnipresent (and well documented in the case of donor conception more broadly, see Becker, Butler & Nachtigall, 2005), the discounting of the genetic contribution made by egg donors has led Martin (2015) to suggest that in some ways surrogacy arrangements evoke a form of neo-eugenics. Taking the genetic materials of another and re-narrating them so that they become one's own (and in so doing discounting their contribution) is, Martin argues, a form of neoeugenics, in that the logic underpinning them is premised upon certain (privileged) groups of people gaining what they want through the discounting of others, by screening for particular traits that are considered to be both genetically determined and desirable, and by instrumentalizing the bodies of certain people in the service of others. Furthermore, and as Martin also notes, surrogacy services are available only to a relatively select few who can afford them. What this means is that whilst for some the stigma of childlessness is mitigated, for others it is compounded.

In this section we have made perhaps some of the strongest claims thus far in this book. We have signalled what Martin (2015) refers to as a 'genetic imperative', and have suggested that it has served to marginalize families, such as those formed through adoption or fostering, in favour of those who can claim some form of genetic relatedness. In terms of genetic relatedness itself, we have followed others in positioning this as a truth claim that is naturalized, one that cannot be abstracted from the contexts in which genetics are made to matter, yet we have contrarily suggested that genetics are sometimes discounted (specifically with regard to egg donors). This has led us to follow Martin in suggesting that certain aspects of surrogacy services eerily mirror the practice of eugenics, even if we acknowledge that this is unlikely to be the intention of both service providers and intending parents. These strong claims may irk some readers, but we feel it important not only to continue to clearly signal our orientation to the topic of surrogacy, but also to clearly discuss the ways in which surrogacy is rendered intelligible via particularly orientations towards kinship (and particularly where the 'hegemony of the gene' is evident). In the following and final section in this chapter we explore what all of this means for critical health psychology.

Critical health approaches to surrogacy

In her book *Explaining Health and Illness*, Wendy Stainton Rogers (1991) identifies cultural critique as a useful way of understanding constructions of health. A focus on cultural critique, she suggests, enables the development of an approach to understanding 'health in terms of power, status and wealth' (p. 139). Such an approach, we would suggest, lends itself well to the study of surrogacy. As we have elaborated throughout this book thus far, the topic of surrogacy, including how one becomes oriented to it, must centrally be concerned with the differential effects of power and status upon how individual parties are rendered vulnerable within both cultural contexts where reproductivity is privileged, and where surrogacy is practised. Furthermore, and as we argued in the previous section, genetic relatedness, for those who are unable to approximate this norm through reproductive heterosex, is the province of those with the funds necessary to enter into surrogacy arrangements and/or to utilize reproductive technologies. And more broadly, through our orientation to surrogacy as a mode of capitalist re-production, wealth is a central point of inquiry in our approach to the topic.

With these points in mind, then, and following the lead set by Stainton Rogers (1991), our understanding of critical health approaches within this book as they pertain to surrogacy takes as its central focus the disparities that lead certain women to act as surrogates or ovum donors, and other people to commission surrogacy arrangements. As is a hallmark of critical health approaches more broadly, then, this focus shies away from health as an individually constituted set of behaviours or actions, and instead locates individuals within their broader social contexts, through which particular behaviours or actions are rendered intelligible for particular individuals, dependent on their social location (see chapters in Murray, 2014). This approach thus supplements our arguments in the previous chapter with regard to vulnerability and the face of the Other.

Through a critical health lens, vulnerability as it pertains to health signals how, under a capitalist logic, we are all rendered vulnerable to the operations of the market, but how this differentially impacts upon our wellbeing. This is not to say that the stigma of infertility nor what may often be experienced as the stigma of commissioning a surrogacy arrangement are equal to the stigma of carrying a child for another person or the possible physical consequences of gestation and birth. Rather, it is to focus on how these vulnerabilities are produced. To turn towards the face of the Other, then, is to acknowledge that one person's 'healthy subject position' (Riggs, 2005) may be the corollary of another person's marginalization. As Butler (2004) suggests, facing the Other is not about facing oneself first. Rather, it is about looking at the social forces that shape all of our experiences, and through which we are made intelligible.

In the chapters that follow, then, our focus is on drawing out how differences in power, status and wealth shape the lives of the groups we look at – women who act as surrogates, intending parents, and the children born to them – before then considering how both surrogacy agencies and the media and legislators become complicit with or resist certain framings of what are construed as either acceptable or unacceptable health consequences of surrogacy. Whilst in some cases these consequences are tied to health as it is more commonly understood – as an individual matter warranting individual attention – in other cases health pertains more broadly to what kind of society we wish to live in, what type of norms shape our experiences, and how surrogacy allows for a focus on the ways in which the injunction to reproductivity (and women's role in this) is so frequently naturalized.

A critical health approach to surrogacy, then, is one that moves beyond seeing surrogacy as simply a 'reproductive health' matter, or one of 'reproductive rights'. Rather, it starts from an orientation to surrogacy, and health more broadly, that sees health as always already framed by a marketplace in which humans are not the primary focus in and of ourselves. Certainly, as we argued in the previous two sections, genetically related children are precious and priceless objects within a capitalist logic, but this is not necessarily because they are an end in and of themselves. Rather, they are the means to an end that never ends: the re-production of capital. The 'healthy subject', then, who complies with the injunction to reproduce in the service of capital (even if this injunction is framed within the language of individual desire, love and care), is a cog in the wider machinery of capitalism. In the final chapter of this book, however, we open up a space for thinking about kinship beyond the marketplace, in an attempt at applying a critical health approach as an intervention into neoliberalism.

3

WOMEN WHO ACT AS SURROGATES

Overview

In this chapter we consider the experiences of women who act as surrogates, particularly in relation to the way this group of women represent themselves, their motivations, and their conceptualizations of surrogacy. As highlighted in the previous two chapters, research on women who act as surrogates has produced widely varied opinions, including conflicting views on the topic. For example, feminist literature concerning women who act as surrogates has highlighted both the need to focus on agency and choice amongst this group of women, but also the fact that acting as a surrogate can be seen as a form of exploitation or commodification, particularly in relation to commercial surrogacy (Raymond, 1993). As such, exploring the experiences and representations of women who act as surrogates is almost by definition an act of disorientation, in that to date previous literature and analysis has refused to present a singular account of the experiences of such women.

In Chapters 1 and 2 we provided an outline of vulnerability as a potential framework for considering all parties in surrogacy arrangements. In relation to women who act as surrogates specifically, there is a relatively large body of literature which recognizes the vulnerability of women who act as surrogates, including feminist literature which has long provided a critical examination of the practice of surrogacy in terms of the potential for exploitation of women acting as surrogates. As Amrita Pande (2011) argues in relation to commercial surrogacy specifically: 'Existing scholarship has convincingly established that commercial surrogacy is culturally disruptive, morally ambiguous and potentially exploitative' (p. 623). This literature mirrors other feminist writing concerning the vulnerabilities of all women in terms of their presumed reproductive capabilities and the subjugating effects this can have (Jones, 1990; Orloff, 1993).

In terms of commercial surrogacy, commentators have highlighted the vulnerability of women who act as surrogates particularly in terms of their potentially limited alternative financial options (see Vora, 2009; Damelio & Sorenson, 2008), arguing that if women who act as surrogates in countries such as India had alternative work options, they would be less likely to choose surrogacy as an option for making money. For example, it has been pointed out that Indian women who act as surrogates can earn the equivalent of 6–10 years' salary acting as a surrogate, thus raising questions about the extent to which acting as a surrogate is truly a choice for Indian women (Haworth, 2007; Blyth, 2008). Vulnerability in this way, then, is conceived of both in terms of the commodification of women's bodies (that is, that the capability of women's bodies for reproduction renders them vulnerable to practices such as surrogacy), as well as inequalities in terms of outcomes and choice between the privileged and the disadvantaged, leading to the potential for exploitation (Rotabi & Bromfield, 2012; Palattiyil, Blyth, Sidhva & Balakrishnan, 2010).

Despite these concerns, it is important to note that research with women who act as surrogates has also highlighted the ways in which women lay claim to the money they earn, and may therefore stand to benefit from surrogacy arrangements. For example, Pande (2009) argues that by outlining alternative discourses about kinship, the women in her study were able to foreground their central and indispensable role in the birth of the child – and in doing so, also lay claim to some of the money they earned. This is important because, as we shall see below, there are concerns that women who act as surrogates are the subject of exploitation not only from the capitalist structures within which they are seen as goods providing a service, but also from pressures placed upon them by their husbands or other family members to act as a surrogate in order to earn money for the family.

As noted above, the body of literature concerning women who act as surrogates is large, and growing. In this chapter we focus specifically on how women who act as surrogates understand surrogacy and the kinship relationships it potentially involves, as well as how they represent themselves as desirable surrogates, their motivations for becoming a surrogate, and their role in the surrogacy arrangement. In order to do so, we consider data from a documentary – *Google_Baby* – which focuses on the experiences of Indian women who act as surrogates. We then compare this data with advertisements placed by women in North America who are willing to act as surrogates derived from two websites: *All About Surrogacy* and *Surromomsonline*. In analysing these data and providing a comparative analysis of the two data sources, we will provide an overview of how women who act as surrogates are currently positioned in surrogacy arrangements, and we take up the implications of this in further detail in the conclusion of this chapter, and in the final chapter of the book.

Before considering these data, we first turn to an examination of the previous literature concerning the experiences of women who choose to act as surrogates. This body of literature spans the experiences of women in a diverse range of countries, including India, Thailand, North America and the UK, where surrogacy arrangements either are, or have been, legal. We explore the findings of this literature in relation to women's understandings of kinship, and their motivations for, and experiences of, acting as a surrogate. It is important to note that in writing this chapter, we are mindful of the necessity to not generalize the experiences of women from different ethnic, cultural, national or socioeconomic backgrounds, nor to assume that straightforward comparisons between the experiences of diverse groups of women are possible. Instead, we aim to provide an overview of the complex interplay of discourses, representations and experiences relating to women who choose to act as surrogates. We do this in order to provide a greater understanding of their role in surrogacy arrangements, and to engage with debates concerning the ways which women who act as surrogates must represent themselves so as to align with particular values accorded to their roles that require them to situate themselves within particular subject positions. These subject positions and values have ongoing implications for women's health and wellbeing, which we explore in the final chapter of this book.

Accounts of motivations and kinship

Research on the experiences of women who act as surrogates varies depending on the country in which the research was conducted, and therefore in relation to the ethnic or cultural background of the women involved in the arrangement. In this section we explore literature relating to two main areas with regard to women who act as surrogates across a variety of cultural contexts. Specifically, we explore the complex interplay of motivations reported by women who act as surrogates, and we take up discussions of norms concerning acceptable motivations and how they may differ from women's 'real' motivations. We also explore norms of kinship and how surrogacy may disrupt those norms, with women who act as surrogates themselves taking up particular kinship discourses which may best suit their needs in the context of an arrangement which may be otherwise (i.e. absent of kinship discourses) seen as exploitative.

Motivations for women to act as surrogates

Acting as a surrogate can lead to financial gain for women, particularly in the context of commercial surrogacy. In India, for example, women are able to earn approximately ten years' worth of income by acting as a surrogate (Pande, 2009), with financial reasons being cited as a leading motivation by many women who act as surrogates (Karandikar, Gezinski, Carter & Kaloga, 2014). Research with women who act as surrogates in other countries – such as the United States, the United Kingdom and Thailand – has similarly found that financial gain is a leading motivation cited by women who act as surrogates (Van den Akker, 2003; Hibino & Shimazono, 2013). This financial gain clearly raises questions as to the autonomy of women who act as surrogates, in addition to concerns about exploitation as noted above, including in relation to exploitation by husbands or male partners who may force women to act as a surrogate for financial gain (Karandikar et al., 2014; Van den Akker, 2003). In relation to the latter concern, Sharmila Rudrappa (2010) argues that commercial surrogacy in India appears to have arisen precisely in order to overcome critiques of exploitation (by ensuring that women get paid for their labour). Nevertheless, such concerns are shown to be warranted by research which has found that women who act as surrogates often have relatively low levels of education, or are from lower socioeconomic or class statuses. This trend has been found both in the context of India (Pande, 2011; Karandikar et al., 2014), the United Kingdom (Van den Akker, 2003), the United States (Jacobson, 2016) and Thailand (Hibino & Shimazono, 2013).

While financial gain may well be a leading motivation for women, a large body of research highlights that this motivation to participate in a surrogacy arrangement is typically seen as shameful, and is socially unacceptable as a primary reason for acting as a surrogate. As noted previously, in the US context Helen Ragoné (1994) found that surrogates are often screened out from working for clinics if they state that their motivations to act as a surrogate are primarily financial, and Heather Jacobson (2016) notes that many agencies will not work with women on welfare benefits so that money is not seen to be the primary motivation for acting as a surrogate. In the Indian context, undertaking surrogacy for financial purposes has been likened to prostitution (Pande, 2009; Hochschild, 2013). Arlie Hochschild notes that this is particularly salient in the case of women who are seen as motivated primarily by making money, rather than by helping other people, where women who are considered too materialistic are seen as dishonourable. Other literature has highlighted similar findings, and has noted that clinics or agencies encourage women not to see themselves as part of financial contracts, but instead as performing altruistic services, and to see themselves as 'angels' or 'heroes' (Pande, 2011; Roach Anleu, 1992; Ragoné, 1994); representations which we consider more in the analytic section of this chapter.

While financial gain is cited consistently in previous research as a leading reason for being involved in a surrogacy arrangement (despite the social taboos surrounding this motivation), previous research has found differences in non-financial or altruistic motivations provided by women who act as surrogates. For example, in the Israeli context, Elly Teman (2010) notes that women acting as surrogates see themselves as giving a priceless gift to another woman (the intended mother), while at the same time accepting that their motivation in the first place may have been economic. Similar discourses have been found in the United States, where research concerning women who act as surrogates has found that women often report a desire to 'help' as a driving force behind their decision to act as surrogates. Here, financial compensation or payment for surrogacy services is seen as primarily part of a reciprocal relationship between themselves and the intending parents, rather than as financial gain (Berend, 2016; Imrie & Jadva, 2014). For example, Zsuzsa Berend found that on the forums she analysed in the United States, women frequently discussed the fact that their primary motivation was altruistic – such as seeing the joy on intending parents' faces when they held their baby for the first time. However, importantly, the women whose narratives Berend explored also noted that they wouldn't act as a surrogate for free, indicating a sense of reciprocity in their gift and the payments they receive. In relation to such representations of altruism, Pande (2011) argues that '[p]art of the dominance of altruism and gift-giving as an ethical norm in the global north derives from its accepted opposition to commercialism' (p. 620), leading to representations of women who act as surrogates as being gift-giving, pure and untainted by capitalism; representations we will explore further in our analysis below.

While research in the United States, the United Kingdom and Israel has typically found discourses of gift-giving to intending mothers or parents amongst women who act as surrogates, much of the research in the Indian context has found that women acting as surrogates displace some of the 'giving' onto the doctors and other medical professionals (e.g. Vora, 2010), while other research has not found discourses of giving to intending parents in research amongst Indian women at all (e.g. Pande, 2011). In relation to the latter findings, Pande argues that the dominant discourse in her ethnographic research of an Indian surrogacy clinic was that of the ability to give to one's own family, that is, a 'God-given opportunity for poor Indian mothers to serve their family' (p. 623). As such, women in Pande's research shifted the rhetoric of 'giving' from intending parents to their own families. In the Thai context, Yuri Hibino and Yosuke Shimazono (2013) found that women often used the concept of *tan-bun* or merit-making to justify their decision; that is, a desire to help others in order to build merit for any previous transgressions.

In addition to altruistic or financial motivations, Jacobson (2016) specifies that the primary motivational 'push' for women acting as surrogates in her research in the United States came through the birth of what they saw as their last child, with many of the women in her study stating that they loved being pregnant and therefore wished to help others to have a baby (see also Ragoné, 1994). This group of women spoke of the love they had for their own families and children, revealing a desire to share their good fortune with others who were unable to have children themselves. Similar findings have been written about in relation to Thailand, with Hibino and Shimazono (2013) finding that women who act as surrogates often cite the fact that they enjoyed being pregnant as a primary motivation to become a surrogate, coupled with the joy of handing the baby to the intended parents. Similarly in the United Kingdom, Imrie and Jadva (2014) also note that the most highly cited motivations in their study were wanting to help others, and enjoying being pregnant.

Overall, the literature suggests various motivations for women who act as surrogates, including potential tensions within these motivations. For example, while financial gain may be a primary motivation in the context of commercial or compensated surrogacy, women also frequently report altruistic motivations such as helping others. Other motivations include personal ones unrelated to financial gain, particularly in relation to enjoyment of being pregnant.

Women who act as surrogates and kinship relations

While kinship has traditionally been considered to be primarily about 'blood lines', recent research – drawing on Schneider's seminal work on the topic (1984) – has highlighted how kinship may in fact be reinterpreted or reconfigured to reflect a diverse and fluid understanding of human relationships (Berend, 2016). In the context of women who act as surrogates, the literature indicates a broad range of differing findings concerning how this extremely heterogeneous group of women view their relationship with the babies they carry, and the parents for whom they carry them. Indeed, differences exist between research findings even in the context of single countries. For example, in the Indian context a body of previous research has found that women discuss creative modes of kinship to draw a link to the baby they carry (Pande, 2009), while other research in the Indian context has found that women deliberately distance themselves from their wombs and the baby inside them (Hochschild, 2013). We discuss these diverse findings in more detail below.

Discourse of kinship and the importance (or lack thereof) of genetic relationships in the context of surrogacy typically differ depending on whether the arrangements are gestational or traditional, and there is a large body of literature in this area. Here we summarize some of the main points as they relate specifically to women who act as surrogates. Jacobson (2016) notes that, essentially, different understandings of kinship are promoted in different surrogacy contexts, in order to ensure that intending parents are seen as the 'rightful' parents of the child, and that their relationship with the child is foregrounded. Specifically, Jacobson notes that genetic bonds are reified in gestational surrogacy, where the baby is seen to be the product of the parents' genetic material, and therefore not related to the women acting as a surrogate at all (although, as we saw in the previous two chapters, such understandings of genetics are simplistic and often incomplete). By contrast, in traditional surrogacy, genetic relationships are frequently played down in favour of intent, such that, again, the intending parents are seen as the rightful parents of the child.

However, despite the presence of discourses which strongly reiterate the primacy of intending parents (often in order to ensure that women acting surrogates will relinquish the baby), Pande (2009) highlights the creative forms of kinship claimed by Indian woman who act as surrogates when they discuss their experiences and relationships to the babies they carry. In her research, Pande discusses how women who act as surrogates place emphasis upon the exchange of bodily substances such as breast milk and blood, and their connection to the child through their shared experiences and the labour that brings them into the world. Pande writes:

> By emphasizing connections based on shared bodily substance and by deemphasizing the ties the baby has with its genetic mother and the men involved in surrogacy (the genetic fathers and the surrogates' husbands), the surrogates challenge established hierarchies in kin relationships – where genes and the male seed triumph above all.
>
> *(2009, p. 380)*

Other research has also highlighted the fluidity of kinship ties through the sharing of bodily substances; ties which are not recognized in dominant discourses of relatedness as connection through biogenetic relationships (e.g. Strathern, 1988; Lambert, 1996). Such dominant discourses tend to privilege the patrilineal relationship between father and child, and thus exploring the experiences and representations of women who act as surrogates is important in relation to disrupting such dominant discourses in order to consider other forms of kinship. Indeed, Pande (2009) argues that while surrogacy and other reproductive technologies are often seen as privileging men's genetic desires (see also Rothman, 1989; Roberts, 1997), the perceptions of Indian women acting as surrogates disrupts this discourse by instead foregrounding other forms of kinship through labour and shared substances.

By contrast, Berend (2016) reports that, in a study of the *Surromomsonline* forum, many of the women who had acted as surrogates did not consider themselves as closely related to the child they carried, with a taken-for-granted stance being that the child would not exist if it weren't for the intending parents. Berend writes that many of the women acting as surrogates on the *Surromomsonline* forum note that in their opinion the baby is not theirs; that they are, in the strict sense, carrying a child for someone else; with the 'social' relationship of the intending parents seen as more important than their own biological relationship. In this sense, the women who act as surrogate and who are members of *Surromomsonline* highlight specifically that 'all' they are doing is providing a uterus – that when the baby is born, they will be giving it back to their parents. Similar findings have been noted by Jacobson (2016) in her study with women in the United States, who similarly stated that they felt they were 'just an oven' (p. 57), and hence downplayed any biological relationship with the child they carried. In this sense, then, they were 'giving babies back rather than giving babies up' (p. 58). As we shall see in Chapter 5, very similar narratives are evoked in children's books that feature narratives of surrogacy.

Research has also extended to consider the ways in which women who act as surrogates express their relationship to the baby they carry. For example, several researchers (e.g. Ragoné, 1999; Baslington, 2002; Van den Akker, 2003) have found that women who act as surrogates typically de-emphasize their genetic link (if they have one) with the child they carry. Similarly, Hochschild (2013) also notes how one of the women acting as a surrogate with whom she spoke stated that she tries to 'detach herself from her baby, her womb, and her clients' (p. 168). Olga Van den Akker argues that this process of detachment or de-emphasis may be a protective mechanism on the part of women acting as surrogates to minimize any potential distress when they hand the baby to his or her intended parents, although she also notes that the women in her research nevertheless did sometimes display distress when they gave birth and handed the baby on (with Jadva, Murray, Lycett, MacCallum & Golombok, 2003, similarly finding that 32 per cent of the women in their study reported experiencing some distress when they handed over the baby).

On the other hand, it should be noted that research with surrogacy clinics in countries such as India has reported that women who may act as surrogates are specifically told that they ought to maintain distance from their clients, their wombs and the baby they carry (Hochschild, 2013). Instructions such as these from clinic directors appear to indicate that such detachment may not be a personal choice but a necessity in a business arrangement. Importantly, however, Hochschild herself notes that the women in the clinic she visited did grieve when they let go the babies they had carried. Other rules and procedures also exist in most agencies and clinics involved in surrogacy to ensure that women acting as surrogates are willing to give up the baby when the time comes, including requirements for women to already have had a baby so that they are more likely to relinquish the baby after birth (Jacobson, 2016; Pande, 2011), and expectations that women have some form of employment or support so that they are not seen to be engaging with surrogacy out of economic necessity (Jacobson, 2016).

This interpretation of surrogacy is also seen in Teman's (2010) book, in which she argues that the women she interviewed also challenged normative understandings of biological relationships, arguing that the women did not necessarily feel connections to the babies they carried. Instead, Teman argues that the women she studied argued that the technologies used to make them pregnant disrupted the 'natural' bond they may otherwise feel for a baby they were pregnant with. In this regard, it is worth noting that there is a body of literature which notes that, rather than develop a relationship with the fetus they are carrying, many women instead speak of developing relationships with intending mothers or parents (Baslington, 2002; Ragoné, 1996). However, such relationships may be hard to maintain – or indeed are discouraged – after the baby is born (Pande, 2011).

Documentary and advertisement analysis

In this section, we explore the experiences of women who act as surrogates in India and women who act as surrogates in North America. In relation to the first group of women, we analyse data from *Google_Baby*, a documentary following the experiences of women in India and the story of a man who, after his own experiences with surrogacy in the United States, explores the option of starting a company which involves creating embryos in the United States, transferring them to India, and implanting them in Indian women. As noted by the man – Doron – himself, the need for this business is based on the desires of intending parents to have Caucasian egg donors, combined with cheaper costs of the surrogacy arrangement in India itself. While India no longer has legal surrogacy clinics such as the one in *Google_Baby*, there are currently similar models in other countries, and thus this documentary provides insight into the experiences of women in situations such as India.

In this section we also explore classified advertisements placed by women choosing to act as surrogates in the United States – namely *All About Surrogacy* and *Surromomsonline*. Previous research exploring *Surromomsonline* has found several main themes, specifically: idealization of the pre-pregnancy lifestyle (a focus on health claims, age, lifestyle), lifestyle choices (abstinence, exercise), cost of surrogacy services, and personal disclosure of various aspects of the woman's life (May & Tenzek, 2011). In our analysis here we aim to build on this previous research in order to compare these data with the representations seen in *Google_Baby*. Taken together, these two sources of data provide us with insight as to how women choosing to act as surrogates represent themselves, as well as the differences which might exist for women in different cultural contexts.

The 'good' surrogate: being humble, compliant and religious

Echoing previous research by Berend (2016) and Rudrappa (2010), *Google_Baby* highlights how women who act as surrogates in India are represented as being 'good' women, despite concerns some intending parents may have about their class or religion (Pande, 2009). For example, in an advertisement for a clinic played on *Google_Baby*, a clinic director notes that:

> All of my surrogates are very humble, simple, nice females. They are very committed, they are very dedicated. They are very religious. They want to do their job in a very dedicated manner. These surrogates, I insist, and they always deliver under my care and supervision.

Similarly, advertisements placed by women wishing to be surrogates in the United States also typically highlight their 'good' characteristics, particularly in relation to having previous children, being willing to travel and – most often – their desire to help other people have a baby. For example:

> Hello I am a 23 year old mother. And would like to become a surrogate for someone. I have read a lot of stories. It's heart breaking to see people out there that can't create their own families. I have a passion for giving. And would love to give the 'gift of life' to someone that cant do it alone.
>
> *('Wanting to help', Surromomsonline)*

> Hi, I'm Marie! I have kids, always thankful to God … I've a part-time job for Business Administration-Marketing, and enjoying life as it comes. I've thought about helping couples have children for years. I have maternal pregnancy cravings. I want to help families have babies because I know how badly I wanted my own children. Now, I have been blessed and working towards a wonderful future with my family. I enjoyed my pregnancies, they were both uncomplicated and healthy pregnancies/vaginal deliveries. I have no health issues. I am 5'7" and weigh 110 lbs. I am negotiable on comp/travel and insurance. Any questions, feel free to ask.
>
> *('Healthy female looking to help couple', All About Surrogacy)*

While the ads from women in the United States did not typically use the word 'humble' (although a minority did), they similarly outline characteristics which suggest that women who act as surrogates should be 'good' and ready to comply with the wishes of intending parents at all times – including in relation to abortion if requested. Indeed, many of the advertisements specifically stated that the woman were happy to abort, particularly up to twenty weeks' gestation. Of note is the fact that the women also frequently discussed issues relating to insurance and health, indicating an awareness of the impact of these issues for intending parents and the potential pregnancy.

Both the advertisements on the two websites and the statement of the clinic director in *Google_Baby* above highlight the importance of religion, with both sources of data frequently discussing religion when advertising their services. Again, this points to the theme of the need to be seen as a 'good' surrogate – religious, humble, compliant and ready to conform to the wishes of intending parents. Of note is the fact that being religious and being prepared to abort a fetus may raise some issues for both women acting as surrogates and intending parents, and indeed one advertisement on *All About Surrogacy* specifically states that the woman is not prepared to abort due to her religion:

> Hello! I'm a first time gestational surrogate looking to help a family out in need. I have three children. I am 22 years old. I live in Pennsylvania. I have been approved medically to do this but I am having trouble finding a couple due to my reasons not to abort. I am a Christian and I believe all life is precious. I desperately want to help out a heterosexual married couple that want a baby. My heart goes out to all of the heart broken couples out there not able to have kids.
>
> *('22 year old ready to be a surrogate', All About Surrogacy)*

Here, the woman in question states that she is having trouble finding intending parents due to her desire not to abort on request. In *Google_Baby*, the women's views on abortion are not shown. However, we do see Doron struggling with the decision to implant two women for one client, in order to ensure a successful pregnancy. While we hear that the client in question is happy to have two babies if both pregnancies are successful, the question is posed as to whether a so-called 'reduction' could be performed if one or both women become pregnant with twins. The phone call we observe ends with an agreement to a reduction, but afterwards Doron notes that it is not a decision he is comfortable with. We do not see the opinions of women themselves, but the impression given is that this would not be something they can choose to agree or disagree with. As such, again, both the advertisements and *Google_Baby* highlight the desirability of a compliant woman when choosing a surrogate, and the need for women wishing to act as surrogates to present themselves as such, even if some compliance may place them in conflict with their religious beliefs.

While the surrogacy advertisements do not provide insight into the specific experiences of women acting as surrogates, *Google_Baby* shows the journey of one woman, through to her caesarean and the moment when she gives the baby to the intending parents. The woman states: 'I will be happy in front of them when I give the baby. No-one will know that I'm giving this child with a pain in my heart. I will make myself happy and give up this baby.' This extract echoes the work of others, including the work of Jadva and colleagues (2003) in the United Kingdom, and Hochschild (2013) in India. Indeed, Hochschild cites a woman saying: 'we will remember these babies for as long as we live' (p. 172). While there have been other stories of women not wishing to give up the child they carried to intending parents (e.g. Van den Akker, 2003), it is clear that the advertisements for women wishing to act as surrogates place great emphasis on their compliance and willingness to act according to the wishes of the intending parents. Arguably, this willingness is also a necessity of becoming a surrogate in India, and thus it is notable that the clear sadness many women experience upon handing over their baby is kept secret and dismissed.

Being 'successful': healthy behaviours and miscarriage

In addition to being humble, compliant and religious, both the forums and *Google_Baby* place great emphasis upon the need to make sure that the pregnancy is 'successful', and therefore that women who act as surrogates are healthy and unlikely to miscarry. As such, women acting as surrogates also represented themselves as healthy and as able to carry a baby to full-term. For example, in *Google_Baby*, a woman describes how she had a miscarriage, following a scene in which she discusses with the clinic director how it might be hard for her to get the payment she wants due to the miscarriage:

> I put my hands on my stomach and felt empty. I was very sad. I have never felt so bad in my life, at that time. That was the worst moment in my life. I really feel bad that I had a miscarriage at 5 months. If I did not miscarry … I don't have a house. I would have bought a house with the money I got and saved some money for my son's future. Now I am working at the surrogate house for a small salary. But for my children's better future, I will try once again to be a surrogate.

As seen in this extract from the documentary, women who have previously had a miscarriage may find it hard to obtain the same level of payment as other women who have experienced healthy and uncomplicated pregnancies and deliveries. Of course, given the prevalence of miscarriage and the fact that it is often unrelated to the potential viability of subsequent pregnancies, this focus on delivery of a healthy baby perhaps suggests more about perceptions of 'good' women who act as surrogates than it does about actual medical motivations on the part of intending parents.

Importantly, the desirability of not having miscarried previously was not confined to *Google_Baby*. The surrogacy forums also included a focus on previous pregnancy history, including stating 'no previous abortions'. However, here, miscarriages were listed as one of many other health-related pieces of information. For example:

> I have helped the parenting dreams of two families come true and would like to help a third, and most likely final, beautiful child come into this world and into your arms.
>
> Hx [History]:
>
> No abortions or miscarriages.
>
> I have 2 daughters born vaginally full term, no meds.
>
> Healthy lifestyle, full time employment. Measure 5'8" and 145lbs. I deliver IN a hospital. My current OB provided care through both surrogacies.
>
> Surrogacies:
>
> Baby A born 7/2013 to adoring daddies. Full term, vaginal birth. Transferred 2 embryos, first transfer success with singleton.
>
> Baby E born 3/2015 to adoring mom/dad. Full term, vaginal birth. Transferred 1 embryo, first transfer successful.
>
> Details:
>
> SET [single embryo transfer] only. Willing to abort up to 20 weeks.
>
> *('Experienced surrogate', Surromomsonline)*

Advertisements with this level of detail were the norm, with others also providing details such as about family relationships (e.g. 'loving'; 'warm'; 'husband with a good sense of humour') and workplaces. As such, we argue that the advertisements on the surrogacy forums demonstrate that it is seen as desirable for potential surrogates to be healthy. As can be seen in the example above, women frequently stated their Body Mass Index (BMI) and other health-related behaviours, as well as listing their previous successful pregnancies and births. In *Google_Baby*, we see a similar focus on health for women acting as surrogates, including scenes where the clinic director imparts information to potential intending parents about women's previous successful pregnancies or surrogacy experiences. In addition, in the Indian context, women who act as surrogates were frequently required to stay within the clinic for the term of their pregnancy, with *Google_Baby* outlining how groups of women shared dormitory-like accommodation for the term of their pregnancy, and were schooled in looking after themselves, resting, and eating healthy food under supervision.

This finding is thus reflective of the previous work by May and Tenzek (2011), which similarly found an emphasis on health and lifestyle choices in their analysis of *Surromomsonline*. As we shall see in Chapter 4, intending parents who advertise on website forums similarly make demands about the health of potential surrogates.

Women's motivations: love or money

Despite our emphasis in the previous sections on women's claims to focusing on the needs of intending parents through being seen as humble, compliant, religious and healthy, the desires (or at least the socioculturally intelligible desires) of women acting as surrogates themselves were evident in both the forums and *Google_Baby*. Notably, these desires are arguably dichotomous: love or money.

In the documentary we see how money can be a driving focus for women who act as surrogates and their families. For example, in one scene, a woman's husband answers questions as to why they want to do surrogacy, stating that they don't have a house and would like to buy one. Moreover, and as noted by Pande (2010), *Google_Baby* also shows how surrogacy can lead to benefits specifically for women, with one scene in which the director of the surrogacy clinic specifies to the woman who acted as a surrogate and her husband that the house they wish to purchase with the money earned from the surrogacy arrangement must be placed in the woman's name alone. The same couple also discuss the opportunities afforded to their son through the money earned in the surrogacy arrangement, thereby reflecting Pande's (2011) findings related to discourses of surrogacy as an opportunity for women in India to serve their families. Thus, money appears to be a key motivation for women in India – albeit often with the desire to help their family as a result of the income they earn.

By contrast, the drive to enter into a surrogacy arrangement in order to make money is not a defining feature of the advertisements on the forums we examined. Instead, the overwhelming theme of the forums we analysed was that of helping others:

> I was on here not long ago and found an amazing IM [intending mother]. We proceeded and I went through contract but unfortunately her little embryos are not passing screening. Sadly I am ready to move on to try and help another family try and achieve their own little family. I am doing this because I truly feel God has blessed my family so much and I would love to give back by helping another family. I hope I can find a couple who is as loving and beautiful as the last couple I found on here. The only thing we will not do is termination, so if that is something you would want in contract we are not the GC for you. Other than that we are okay with transferring two embryos and just hope we can find two loving people who want to start a family! God Bless, we look forward to hearing from you.
>
> *('Surrogate looking for good match', Surromomsonline)*

> My name is Bria I am 22, engaged, and have 1 child of my own and now I can appreciate the joy of being a parent and would love to help someone experience the feeling as well. Being a surrogate to help a family grow has always been a passion in my heart.
>
> *('Mum wishing to be a surrogate for the first time', All About Surrogacy)*

A common thread in these posts was the drive to help others after experiencing the joy of being a parent oneself. Moreover, some people specifically stated that their motivations were not financial. As one woman stated: 'I am not doing this for the money but rather the joy of helping someone to have a baby of they're [*sic*] own.' Other women noted that they do not wish to organize the surrogacy arrangement through an agency as they are clear that they are not out to make money, but rather to help intending parents. Clearly, it is not possible to ascertain women's primary motivations through the advertisements on surrogacy forums. Nevertheless, and as noted by others (Rudrappa, 2010), it would appear evident that a primary desirable characteristic of a woman wishing to act as a surrogate is that their motivations are altruistic (even in the case of commercial surrogacy) and not related to financial gain. This is also seen in *Google_Baby* in relation to the advertisement from the clinic which specifies, as noted above, that women acting as surrogates through the clinic are dedicated, humble and religious.

As we will argue in the following chapter, the binary of love or money is complicated in the context of surrogacy, as Zelizer (2005) suggests it is in neoliberal societies more broadly. Whilst we have suggested that the monetary aspects of surrogacy appear more salient in the Indian context as compared to the US contexts (where the women advertising on the websites were located), it is too simplistic to suggest that this indicates a fundamental difference in how love or money shape women's experiences in the two contexts, absent from consideration of the broader social forces at work. In other words, differences between the two countries may arguably produce either love or money as the most salient factors, dependent on, for example, the degree of social welfare available, public discourses about women's role in society, and the location of each country within broader global forces. Moreover, the overt focus on love rather than money in the online forums may also reflect desirable characteristics for women acting as surrogates from the perspective of the intending parents. Nevertheless, this dichotomy is interesting for what it tells us about the identities which women wishing to act as surrogates must portray, and therefore how surrogacy itself is placed in a broader sociocultural context.

Agency and shame

While the previous sections detail some potential differences in the representations and motivations of women acting as surrogates depending on the sociocultural context, our analysis of forums and *Google_Baby* indicated that there were two further large differences in terms of the representations of the experiences of women acting as surrogates: agency and shame.

In relation to shame, *Google_Baby* provides an overview of the secrecy which women who act as surrogates in India must adhere to. As one interviewee stated: 'No-one knows I am a surrogate except my husband. I have told everyone that I am going to America to earn some money.' Later, we see the clinic director speak to this woman after the baby is delivered, reiterating that she must not tell others about her experiences acting as a surrogate. In another scene, a woman working at the clinic outlines the main cause of the secrecy:

> Some surrogate mothers tell to parents they are doing a surrogate mother. And some are not telling. And in a very conservative society where she doesn't know how people will look at them, there are people who compare it to prostitution.

Previous literature also indicates that women acting as surrogates in India are often required to hide their involvement in a surrogacy arrangement, particularly due to comparisons with prostitution. Hochschild (2013), for example, notes how one of the women in her study moved her family to another village in order to hide the fact that she was acting as a surrogate, and similar situations have been documented in other research (Rudrappa, 2010; Haworth, 2007). The advertisements on the two websites we considered for this chapter display no similar evidence of secrecy in relation to surrogacy.

In relation to the second issue of agency, and as noted previously, women acting as surrogates in the Indian context were strictly supervised and monitored for the duration of their pregnancy, living in dormitories in surrogacy clinics with other women. Pande (2009) notes in her research that the women she spoke to frequently formed strong bonds with the other women in the clinic, and while this is also seen in the documentary, *Google_Baby* also discusses the hardships that living in dormitories brings. For example, as noted by one woman: 'Sometimes they are crying for family. Something's happened – their father is not feeling well or their husband is not feeling well.' In this sense, then, it is arguable that one of the main differences between the likely experiences of women acting as surrogates in the US context as compared to the Indian concept lies in the area of agency. Specifically, women who act as surrogates in India live their lives during their pregnancy under the strict supervision of clinic staff, with little say over their actions and little choice about their medical situations. This is also seen in the two scenes in *Google_Baby*, where women have caesareans to deliver the babies, with women apparently having little choice in relation to issues such as pain relief. Indeed, one scene shows a woman quite distressed at the level of pain she experiences when having a caesarean. The issue of agency also comes to the fore in the scene discussed previously, with Doron negotiating the implantation of two women and potential reduction of fetuses with no consultation with the women involved. While we do not see this play out, it appears reasonable to suggest that these decisions would be made with clinic directors with minimal consultation with the women acting as surrogates themselves.

By contrast, the advertisements placed by potential surrogates on the two forums appear to show high levels of agency for women in the United States. Here, we see women frequently specifying particular conditions relating to their pregnancy, although, and in line with the first theme above, their dominant representation of themselves was as humble and ready to 'help'. For example, while we noted above that it was typical for women to state that they were prepared to abort fetuses, a smaller number of advertisements did specify that the women involved would not have an abortion unless it was medically indicated, suggesting that there is a degree of autonomy and agency for women acting as surrogates in the United States, at least in relation to some of the choices about how their bodies are used. For example:

> I want to help carry for a family because everyone deserves the chance to have a child. I'm opposed to abortion for any reason, multiples if unwanted will not be terminated. Insurance will be needed. I don't mind gay couples at all. I just want to give what I've been blessed with.
>
> (*'Healthy surrogate ready to help family', Surromomsonline*)

Again, issues of agency and shame likely relate closely to specific sociocultural circumstances, including cultural norms concerning the role of women, religion and broader attitudes towards surrogacy in the community. For example, Teman's (2010) research concerning surrogacy in Israel indicates that the women in her study saw themselves as agentic – at least to a certain degree. For example, she cites one of the women she spoke with as specifically stating that she was not a robot, but 'here in order to help' (p. 31). In this sense, then, women who act as surrogates are very much at the mercy of the broader attitudes and norms in their own specific cultural context.

Concluding thoughts

In this chapter we have outlined the sometimes competing themes and discourses surrounding the experiences, motivations and representations of women who act as surrogates in two distinct cultural contexts. Our analysis indicates that there are a range of desirable characteristics and subject positions for women who choose to act as surrogates. In particular, our analysis highlights how women who act as surrogates are required to promote themselves as ready to help intending parents become pregnant, and to present themselves as healthy, compliant and humble. Our analysis also noted some tensions between motivations of love or money for women acting as surrogates, albeit with a degree of overlap in the practical outcomes of these distinct motivations. Finally, we noted differences in the likely experiences of women who choose to act as surrogates, indicating that women are likely at the mercy of broader cultural norms if they do choose to act as a surrogate.

Looking at both the surrogacy forums and *Google_Baby* also enabled us to identify contradictory views in relation to representations of women choosing to act as surrogates – particularly in terms of motivations of love or money. As noted earlier in this chapter, much of the previous research concerning experiences of women who choose to act as surrogates has found discourses of 'gift-giving' or 'helping' as central to the understandings of the motivations of women involved as surrogates, and this was also reflected in our analysis of surrogacy forums. Indeed

– beyond sometimes mentioning insurance – none of the advertisements we analysed on the forums discussed remuneration specifically. Of course, motivations concerning love and money are never clear-cut, as seen in discussions in *Google_Baby* concerning the desire of some of the women portrayed in the documentary to earn money to support family and children. Nevertheless, it is arguable that financial motivations appeared to be downplayed or dismissed in the forums, and justified in *Google_Baby* by reference to the purpose of earning money in relation to supporting family. As argued by Pande (2011): 'Surrogates' devaluation of remuneration … can be understood to fulfil two functions: to reiterate the widely held belief that children are priceless and simultaneously prove that they are "pure" surrogates reproducing for the couple as a "gift"' (p. 621). Indeed, notions of 'purity' also played out in our analysis in relation to religion, health and desire to be seen as humble and compliant, suggesting that being seen as 'pure' was a driving motivation for women in both contexts.

While tensions between love and money as motivations for acting as a surrogate are interesting to explore in terms of what they tell us about surrogacy and the position of women who choose to act as surrogates, it is also notable that women who choose to act as surrogates need to explain their motivations in the first place. In relation to this, Pande (2011) notes that surrogacy falls somewhere between 'contractual dealing and motherly altruism', and is therefore 'culturally anomalous' (p. 621). This anomalous status of surrogacy and therefore women who act as surrogates is arguably evident not only in the tensions we note between love and money, but also in the ways these tensions exist because of the expectation that women choosing to act as surrogates need to justify their wish to be involved in surrogacy. Furthermore, these justifications need to also be read alongside discussion of particular characteristics (being compliant, humble and so forth), which make them desirable to intending parents. In this way, then, women who act as surrogates are required to behave in particular ways which may offset the otherwise anomalous nature of surrogacy: and in particular, they are required to behave in ways which can be read as consistent with cultural norms concerning 'good' women.

In the first two chapters of this book we discussed how specific women's bodies are commodified through a series of practices that produce women's bodies as viable producers of goods. Indeed, through these understandings, certain women's bodies can be seen as becoming goods in and of themselves. This representation of some women's bodies as viable producers of goods was seen in our analysis of the two sources of data, particularly through a focus on women's health and their previous pregnancy history. Here, women's bodies were only seen as viable for surrogacy if they met particular criteria – including some criteria (e.g. history of miscarriage) that may have little impact on subsequent pregnancies. As such, we argue that specific bodies become desirable for surrogacy and for carrying a child – with this set of criteria arguably creating the conditions for women who act as surrogates to be seen primarily as good, which can serve a function, rather than people in and of their own right.

There was also a sense in the data – specifically with regard to the intelligible subject positions made available to, or taken up by, women who act as surrogates – that certain subject positions more readily allow for the fantasy of oneness to be achieved by intending parents. A compliant, willing 'vessel' is an ideal route through which intending parents can enact their desire for a child 'of their making'. This is not to suggest that women who act as surrogates may not be agentic, and certainly not to confirm that they are in fact empty vessels. Rather, it is to highlight that in taking up these types of subject positions, women who act as surrogates are potentially doing so because such subject positions neatly accord with the broader aims of surrogacy arrangements: to emulate reproductive heterosex. Indeed, that many women who act as surrogates seek to enjoy a relationship with intending parents, but that such a relationship most often disappears after the birth of a child, suggests that any relationship established during the pregnancy may be part of a broader desire to claim the pregnancy, rather than per se to develop a relationship with the woman carrying the child. This is a concern that we explore in more detail in the following chapter, where we turn to focus on intending parents.

4

INTENDING PARENTS

Overview

In this second analytic chapter we focus on intending parents who commission surrogacy arrangements. As was the case in Chapter 3, we do not provide an overview of the entire body of literature that has focused on intending parents. Rather, we focus on two specific topics that have received considerable attention within the literature, both of which arguably demonstrate many of our concerns with regards to the operations of capitalism, the production of vulnerability, and claims to agency through the assumption of intent, as outlined in Chapter 1.

The first of the topics we focus on explores how intending parents initially negotiate surrogacy arrangements, and specifically how they advertise, with the aim of identifying a woman who may act as a surrogate for them. In their work on the topic of surrogacy, Charlotte Kroløkke and Saumya Pant (2012) coin the term 'repropreneurs' to refer to people who draw upon neoliberal discourses in order to warrant their reproductive decisions and actions. Specifically, and as the term would suggest, the repropreneur is a reproductive entrepreneur, or as Kroløkke and Pant suggest, someone who sees themselves as a 'pioneer' in terms of reproduction. This suggestion mirrors that made by Rudrappa (2015) in her claim that intending parents may see themselves as 'moral pioneers' (p. 7) creating new futures and new forms of kinship. In their advertisements, and as we demonstrate below, intending parents position themselves as active agents of neoliberalism, negotiating for their desires to be met, and doing so in ways that both affirm their location within a normative understanding of kinship, whilst nonetheless drawing on the language of consumption through which to authorize their actions.

The second topic we focus on pertains to the ways in which intending parents lay claim to the pregnancies that they commission as their own. As we shall see in our analysis below, not only do heterosexual women make these claims, but so too often do gay men. Such constructions of the surrogate pregnancy function, we suggest, to minimize the repropreneurship that appears evident in the advertisements that intending parents place, instead emphasizing the naturalness of the surrogacy arrangements as a fulfilment of a reproductive destiny centred upon the love for a child. As such, whilst advertising for a surrogacy arrangement represents an obvious form of capitalism at work, claiming the subsequent pregnancy as one's own functions to minimize or deny the capitalist logic at play. Furthermore, and as we argue, what disappears are the bodies of women who act as surrogates, as does the vulnerability that intending parents potentially experience due to being positioned as failed (i.e. infertile) reproductive citizens.

In order to illustrate these claims we analyse two different data sources. The first of these are advertisements placed by intending parents on one of two websites: *All About Surrogacy* and *Surromomsonline*. Both of these websites provide forums in which intending parents, women willing to act as surrogates, and people willing to act as gamete donors, can make listings. In this chapter we specifically focus on intending parents (or their representatives in the form of fertility clinics) and their advertisements as available on the websites in the first four months of 2016. These websites are open to the general public, and do not require a subscription through which to view the advertisements. Our analysis of claims by intending parents about the pregnancy is based upon five self-help books written by parents who had children through surrogacy: four gay couples and one heterosexual couple. The books are: *Dads: A Gay Couple's Surrogacy Journey in India* (Hirschi, 2014), *A Gay Couple's Journey Through Surrogacy: Intended Fathers* (Menichiello, 2012), *The Journey of Same-Sex Surrogacy: Discovering Ultimate Joy* (Warner, 2013), *Our 'Journey': One Couple's Guide to US Surrogacy* (Westoby, 2013) and *Baby Ava: An Irish Surrogacy Story* (O'Flaherty & O'Flaherty, 2012). Before presenting our analysis of these data, however, we first turn to consider what has previously been written in the academic literature on the topics of advertising for surrogacy arrangements and the claiming of pregnancies by intending parents.

Advertising for surrogacy arrangements

Previous literature that has focused on how intending parents make decisions about surrogacy arrangements typically brings together two areas that, as we argued in Chapter 1, are seen as distinct: love and money. Yet following Zelizer (2005), as many working in the field of surrogacy have done (e.g. Dempsey, 2014), it can be argued that love and money are thoroughly intertwined with one another in capitalist societies. Indeed, we are reminded here of Lacan's argument about the problematic of 'your money or your life'. As Lacan argues, this is a false choice as a life without money is a difficult life, just as there is little point in having money if you cannot enjoy your life (Riggs, 2015a). With regard to our orientation to capitalism, then, finance, transactions and love are part and parcel of the one logic, not simply with regard to surrogacy but in neoliberal societies more broadly.

Whilst our claims above, following Zelizer (2005), hold true across multiple relationship and kinship forms, they are perhaps especially true in the context of surrogacy. For intending parents, this gives rise to a complex series of negotiations over the extent to which women who act as surrogates should do so out of care or altruism (what we referred to in Chapter 2 as a properly gendered orientation), but that at the same time payment is important as it allows for the intent (and payment) of the intending parents to become the most rightful claim to the child who is born. Kroløkke and Pant's use of the term 'repropreneur' again usefully highlights how reproduction in the context of surrogacy becomes the province of enterprising individuals who are able to negotiate the neoliberal marketplace in order to achieve what they desire: a child.

In her research with Israeli heterosexual couples entering into surrogacy arrangements, Teman (2010) suggests that the discourse of entrepreneurship is specifically gendered, with men more likely than women to reduce surrogacy arrangements to business deals. This, however, might have been specific to Teman's sample, or the cultural context in which her research was undertaken. In Israel – where pronatalism is explicitly state-sponsored, and where intending mothers are treated as the pregnant person, not the women acting as a surrogate – it is perhaps understandable that Israeli women are less likely to evoke an understanding of surrogacy as a business arrangement. Israeli men, by comparison, may be more likely to be somewhat divorced from the procedure, and to focus primarily on the costs.

In other contexts, however, women may be equally likely to focus on their skills as repropreneurs able to negotiate surrogacy arrangements. Amy Speier (2011), for example, suggests that the women in her sample spoke about 'doing the research' (p. 594), which involved lengthy investigations of clinics, travel details, clinical procedures and likely outcomes. This is not to suggest that love was not also a factor driving the women in their investigations, but that their role as agentic reproductive citizens largely shaped the ways in which they narrated their capacity to negotiate travelling in order to access services.

When it comes to searching for a woman who will act as a surrogate, the work of the repropreneur becomes perhaps most visible. This is someone who not only can 'do the research', but who can also know what they should be looking for, and how to market themselves so that they will be appealing to a potential surrogate. Deborah Dempsey's (2014) research with gay men negotiating surrogacy arrangements suggests that such men 'described the process of selecting their anonymous egg donor as involving a spreadsheet and a list of criteria, comparing it to the process they used to buy their house' (p. 274). Whilst Dempsey's focus in this instance was on egg donors, as we shall see in our analysis below, a similar form of accounting is utilized by intending parents advertising for women who will act as surrogates.

Yet it is not simply the case that intending parents have lists outlining what they are looking for in regards to women willing to act as surrogates. They also display awareness of how to best position themselves so as to attract such women. In their analysis of one of the websites that we too will examine below, Amy May and Kelly Tenzek (2016) suggest that intending parents

> Proactively use disclosure in online ads, revealing intimate details of their relationships, their struggles to complete the parenthood journey, and personal thoughts and feelings in an attempt to reduce uncertainty and facilitate the matching process with a surrogate … [claims to] stability function as a communicative strategy to reduce uncertainty by making readers aware of how they have set up their life to be ready for parenthood, thus eliminating anxieties related to delivering a child into an unprepared family.
>
> *(pp. 6, 8)*

Rudrappa (2014) too, in her examination of how gay men who have had children through surrogacy represent themselves on blogs, suggests that self-representations of competency, stability and parental accomplishments serve to position intending parents as successful repropreneurs. As these examples suggest, whilst it is certainly the case that narratives of love (often in the form of parental competency) frequently appear in advertisements or other materials in which intending parents depict themselves to others, such narratives primarily appear to function to shore up an account of intending parents as agentic repropreneurs.

In his research with gay men who had undertaken surrogacy arrangements, Murphy (2015) suggests that a focus on the transactional nature of surrogacy often translates into a logic whereby intending parents can 'contract out of social obligations through payment' (p. 181). Interestingly, Murphy goes on to note that whilst payment to egg donors or women who act as surrogates is presumed to sever any ties or claims that women may have to children created from their eggs or carried by them, payment serves to strengthen ties between intending parents and children. The successful repropreneur, then, is someone who is able to successfully market themselves to others, successfully identify the goods that they need to purchase in order to meet their needs, and then to utilize the logic of the marketplace to contract out of any obligations to other parties involved in the arrangement. Whilst this account may sound overly mercenary and critical of intending parents, it highlights how a capitalist logic shapes the ways in which surrogacy is often understood, and also highlights how the vulnerability of intending parents (to the norm of reproductive citizenship, to their reliance on other people to fulfil this demand) is made to disappear through a focus on the operations of the marketplace.

Having contracted out of social obligations, then, the stage is set for intending parents to then stake a claim to the pregnancy itself. Obviously, as we noted above with regard to Teman's research (2010), in some contexts the state actively works to assert the intending mother as the person who is pregnant. Yet even in other contexts where the state does not play such an active role, intending parents make claims to the pregnancy. Rudrappa (2015), for example, focusing on the Indian context, suggests that

> engaging in market relations, then, allowed the clients to eliminate the producer. By eliminating her, they recast her labor effort in pregnancy as theirs.

> And they asserted that they were the baby's true and only parents because this baby existed through their intentions.
>
> *(p. 142)*

Also in the Indian context, Vora (2014) suggests that invitations to intending parents to 'view their embryos under the microscope in the embryology lab before implantation' and subsequent invitations to 'attend a 4D sonography session later in the surrogate's pregnancy' work to 'create intimacy and sociality between the commissioning parents and the fetus [but] simultaneously work to erase the woman acting as the gestational surrogate' (p. 71). Dana Berkowitz and William Marsiglio (2007) similarly suggest that the North American gay men they interviewed who had entered into surrogacy arrangements 'discussed living vicariously through the actual pregnancy' (p. 377). Their interviewees did this by staying in close contact with the woman carrying their child throughout the pregnancy, including attending medical appointments and scheduling regular telephone conversations or emails so as to learn about the progress of the pregnancy.

If we return to our arguments in Chapter 1 about the fantasy of oneness, we can conjecture that when intending parents make claims to the pregnancy they are potentially denying that three or four make one, and instead are asserting that it is only two (i.e. the two intending parents, if it is a couple) who make one. Not only is pregnancy – perhaps especially for women but also for some men – a valorized social role that may be seen as desirable to lay claim to (what Teman, 2010, p. 179, refers to as 'pseudoprocreation'), but in order to fully occupy a place within the norm of reproductive citizenship, a claim to the pregnancy appears to become for some intending parents an essential practice in rewriting their vulnerability as a story of agency and success (Riggs & Due, 2013).

It would be remiss of us, however, not to note the views of women who act as surrogates. Certainly in Teman's (2010) research, many of the women she interviewed appeared to equally insist that the pregnancy was not their own, but was rather that of the intending mother. Teman's participants who had carried a child for someone else engaged in forms of strategic naturalizing by insisting that, given the baby was not created from their body, it was 'unnatural', and hence the pregnancy was not their own. Conversely, however, Amrita Pande's (2009) participants in India denied the suggestion that the pregnancy was not their own, as clearly evidenced in the title of Pande's paper, which quotes from a participant who stated that 'it may be her eggs but it's my blood'. For some of the Indian women she interviewed who had acted as a surrogates, then, the blood of the surrogate body was privileged over the genetic material of the intended mother.

As we have suggested in our review of a selection of the previous literature on intending parents, tensions between love and money play out through the trope of the repropreneur, who successfully negotiates surrogacy arrangements that absolve them of vulnerability, and which to a large degree contract them out of relationships with the woman who carries their child. This then leaves some intending parents, it would seem, free to stake a claim to the pregnancy as their own. We now turn to explore these issues as they appear in our data.

Analysis of advertisements and books

In the sections below we first explore advertisements placed by intending parents seeking a woman to carry a child for them, before then examining how self-help books written by intending parents both remove women who act as surrogates from the equation (primarily by disparaging or discounting their role) before then making a claim to the pregnancy itself.

'Seeking surrogate'

In examining advertisements placed by intending parents on the forums hosted on both *All About Surrogacy* and *Surromomsonline*, a significant number were posted by agencies representing intending parents. Of these 'professionally represented' advertisements, all follow a very clear script. They typically first describe in glowing terms the personal characteristics of the intending parents, often with reference to their love for children, their experiences with children, and their altruistic or humanitarian acts. The advertisements then briefly outline the employment situation of the intending parents, with all having jobs described as prestigious (i.e. lawyers, financiers) and well paid. The advertisements typically close with a statement claiming that 'they [i.e. the intended parents] have the resources to pay you a generous fee in addition to all medical, legal, travel and other expenses'. Whilst these scripts are interesting with regard to what they privilege (i.e. money and prestige), we have chosen not to focus on these in any depth given they have already been addressed in the work of May and Tenzek (2016).

Whilst approximately half of the advertisements on the websites involved intending parents who were professionally represented, half were placed by intending parents representing themselves. These advertisements follow similar scripts, but are typically less effusive in their language, often place greater emphasis on the characteristics required of women who may potentially act as surrogates, more clearly talk about money, and often include narratives about the hardship faced by the intending parents. In the remainder of this section we focus specifically on three aspects of the advertisements that we examined:

1 how the journey to surrogacy is framed;
2 the characteristics required of women who will potentially act as surrogates; and
3 the ways in which compensation is discussed.

With regard to the journey to surrogacy, and different from the professionally represented advertisements (which avoid discussions of hardship, instead focusing on the decision to consider a surrogacy arrangement as a welcomed and celebrated aspect of a parenting journey), advertisements placed by intending parents themselves often emphasized hardship, or reproductive challenges that have led to the need to consider a surrogacy arrangement. For some intending parents, such as in the first two quotes below, specific fertility related issues are mentioned:

> We are a 30-something couple in NJ who has tried on our own to conceive, but realized it's just not going to happen ... My wife is unable to carry a child due to a thin Uterine lining and we've been told a GS is likely the only way we can have a child of our own. This is where we are seeking help.
>
> *('In search of healthy, experienced surrogate', All About Surrogacy)*

> My husband and I are looking for a gestational carrier to help us start our family. We are 31 years old, live in Philadelphia, PA, and have been married for 1.5 years (but together for almost 10). I was diagnosed with breast cancer when I was 29 and am very, very grateful to have survived it. However, my medical treatment prevents me from being able to carry a baby.
>
> *('Looking for: Gestational carrier', Surromomsonline)*

In addition to outlining fertility issues as reasons for 'seeking help', these two advertisements also highlight a number of normative assumptions that often appeared within the sample more broadly. First is the privileging of a 'child of our own'. In the first example fertility issues and the desire to have a child automatically default to considering options that allow for a child genetically related to the parents. Similarly, in the second example the woman's 'medical treatments prevents [her] from being able to a carry a baby', which presumes that the only way to have a child is to either carry one or have someone carry a child for you. Excluded from these types of statements are the potential to adopt a child (or indeed not to have a child at all). A similar drive to having a genetically related child is evident in the following advertisement extract:

> I'm a 36yo straight man living in bay area. all my life all I dreamed of was getting married and having a big family with kids but fate never brought that ONE woman to me who wanted a real big family and kids. so now at 36 my options are getting thinner and thinner and I just cant wait any more to find that special someone in my life in order to date, marry and have kids.
>
> *('In search of: TS', All About Surrogacy)*

Again, adoption appears to be precluded as a potential way of having children. Also evident in this advertisement, and as was the case in a considerable number of advertisements placed by intending parents, it was a traditional surrogacy arrangement ('TS') being sought. A traditional surrogacy arrangement typically involves the fertilization of the woman's own egg. As we know from the case of Baby M, this type of arrangement can often be fraught, and particularly if such arrangements are undertaken outside of clinics (i.e. if home insemination is used, and sperm are not screened prior to insemination). Whilst clearly for this particular intending parent the desire for a child is significant, our concern is with the ways in which such a desire can potentially override consideration of the challenges, consequences and potential implications of entering into traditional surrogacy arrangements.

Turning to consider how women who may potentially act as surrogates are depicted in the advertisements, many of those placed by intending parents themselves outlined relatively strict requirements of women, as can be seen in the following two examples:

> You: Lead a healthy lifestyle, have children on your own, open minded, honest, uncomplicated and ready to embark on this adventure together, experienced surrogate is a plus, with insurance from a surrogate friendly state.
>
> *('In search of: TS near NYC/NJ/PA wanted', All About Surrogacy)*

> We are looking for someone who:
> - Is responsible
> - Has a BMI of 29 or below
> - Has had 2 or fewer C-Sections
> - Has a history of healthy pregnancies
> - Has had fewer than 5 births
> - Will leave medical and termination decisions up to the doctors/IPs
> - Is comfortable transferring multiple embryos if medically indicated.
>
> *('Looking for: Gestational carrier', Surromomsonline)*

The first of these examples is arguably more approachable than the second, though nonetheless places a series of demands upon women who may potentially act as a surrogate for the couple, specifically to be 'uncomplicated' and to have their own insurance. This is potentially unrealistic to expect of any private surrogacy arrangement, as it places a considerable burden upon women to have their own insurance (rather than all expenses being covered by the intending parents). The requirement to have their own insurance appeared in many of the advertisements placed by intending parents themselves. The second example above takes the form of a list, and such lists appeared in many of the advertisements that we examined. Some of the items on the list would be typical requirements of an agency recruiting women to act as surrogates (i.e. pregnancy history), whilst others are much more subjective, and indeed regulatory demands (i.e. to be 'responsible'). The demand to concede control over terminations or the number of embryos transferred constitutes a significant potential demand, and we would suggest reflects the framing of the advertisement as 'looking for a gestational carrier', which potentially reduces women's bodies to vessels that can be controlled by others.

Finally, with regard to the advertisements placed by intending parents, money was often discussed in ways that clearly stated that the intending parents could not afford to provide high levels of compensation, as can be seen in the following two examples:

> We aren't rich – I'm an actor and my husband works for an educational non-profit. We were hoping to pay our surrogate $10,000 as well as travel costs, medical costs, legal fees, and any other expenses associates with the pregnancy. Our first surrogate used her own health insurance to cover the pregnancy itself, and we're hoping for a repeat of that arrangement.
>
> (*'In search of: GS – gay couple in Chicago'*, *All About Surrogacy*)

> I have been trying to have a baby for a long time. Please keep in mind, while I would love to pay you a high rate of compensation for the gift of finally granting me the baby I have been longing for, I am looking for someone who is seeking reasonable compensation.
>
> (*'Looking for: Gestational/traditional surro California'*, *Surromomsonline*)

In the first example, and different to the professionally represented advertisements, the intending parents are depicted as not being rich. Echoing the requirements of women who will potentially act as surrogates outlined with regard to one of the extracts above, the intending parents here also indicate that the woman should have her own insurance, and use the example of a previous surrogacy arrangement to authorize this request. The second example above combines an implicit claim to not having funds (i.e. 'trying to have a baby for a long time' implies that the person has already spent a lot of money and may have little left), with the suggestion that acting as a surrogate is 'the gift of finally granting me the baby I have been longing for'. The evocation of the language of a 'gift' potentially serves to mitigate the 'reasonable compensation' being offered (i.e. one does not typically expect payment when one gives a gift). Other advertisements made further claims that appear to mitigate the low compensation being offered, as can be seen in the following two examples:

> We have been through a lot in the last couple years trying to build our family so we cannot afford thousands of dollars. We are looking for a low comp GC who would want to establish friendship with our family and the new baby. A health insurance without surrogacy exclusion would be a plus.
>
> (*'In search of: A gestational surrogate'*, *All About Surrogacy*)

> We are a one income family. The comp we could afford would be for clothes, and medical co-payments. We're really looking for someone to do this not for financial reasons but for helping us complete our family.
>
> (*'Seeking: We want to complete our family'*, *All About Surrogacy*)

In both of these examples women who may potentially act as surrogates are invited into a 'helping' relationship or 'friendship' with the intending parents. Again, this type of language offsets the offer of minimal compensation by suggesting that the benefits of acting as a surrogate are not primarily financial, but rather are about caring relationships. Whilst this might well be a genuine claim on the part of the intending parents, previous research has suggested that once children are born, intending parents typically distance themselves from the woman who carried their child for them (e.g. Ragoné, 1994; Teman, 2010).

In this section we have indicated three key themes that appear in the advertisements we examined. First, the implied desire for genetic relatedness seems to lead to surrogacy as the default option for having a child if one of the intending parents cannot carry the child. Second, demands placed upon women who may act as surrogates serve to reduce them to objects. And third, claims to a gift or caring relationship between women who act as surrogates and intending parents are seen as mitigating the need for adequate compensation. All three of these themes emphasize the tensions between love and money: on the one hand these are arrangements shaped by capitalism, involving the exchange of goods for money, and none of the advertisements easily escape this logic, no matter the language used. On the other hand, however, love becomes a reason to want a child through surrogacy, and then a reason for a woman to act as a surrogate. As we shall see in the following section, however, once surrogacy arrangements are negotiated, there appears to be something of a shift in terms of the distribution of the love component between the parties.

Removing surrogates from the equation

Whilst surrogate arrangements integrally involve a woman willing to carry a child for another person/s, as we suggested in the previous section it would appear that advertisements placed by intending parents appear, at least in many cases, to foreshadow the ways in which women may subsequently be marginalized or excluded from the family. Certainly in some of the advertisements we examined, including the final two examples included in the previous section, the intending parents expressed a desire to develop an ongoing relationship with the woman who carries a child for them. However, largely across the literature on surrogacy it would appear that once the child is born, intending parents distance themselves from the woman who carried their child. In this section we consider how intending parents retrospectively provide examples of how they distanced themselves, or warranted such distancing, including during the pregnancy.

The self-help books written by intending parents that we consider in both this section and the following cover a myriad of topics, include the journey to (and reasons for) surrogacy, challenges in finding a woman willing to carry a child, the intricacies of achieving a pregnancy, the pregnancy itself, and life after the child is born. Given the diversity of these topics, we cannot examine all of them in detail sufficient enough to adequately attend to their complexity. Instead, we focus solely on chapters that discuss the pregnancy itself.

In terms of distancing strategies, three of the books spend considerable portions of their chapter/s on pregnancy discussing how challenging the authors found their relationship with the women who carried a child for them. It is of course understandable that, as with any relationship, stress may at times place individuals in antagonistic relationships with one another. Yet the extracts included below, it is argued here, go beyond the simple expression of antagonism in a stressful situation, and extend to the depiction of women who act as surrogates as troubling impositions upon the lives of the intending parents.

In the text that preceded the first extract below, the author had reported that the woman who was acting as the surrogate – who was a friend of the author – had expressed a desire for a vaginal birth. The author then went on to say, however, that:

> In all honesty, we really would have preferred for her to have agreed up front to have a C-section. Not because we are 'too posh to push', but because it would enable us to plan all of the logistics around when the children were going to be born.
>
> *(Westoby, 2013, n.p.)*

Putting aside the rather odd comment about not being 'too posh to push' (given this claim is normally made about women's decisions in relation to their own bodies, not about men's decisions or bodies), the author's seemingly mundane emphasis upon wanting to 'plan all of the logistics' is perhaps rather less mundane if we consider the position of the men, who do not have full 'access' to their child until s/he is born. Indeed, it is one thing for two men to wish to 'plan all of the logistics' related to the birth of a child, but it is another thing altogether to be the woman who is giving birth, for whom logistics may be just one of many concerns. Reducing the pregnancy and birth (and thus the woman undertaking both) to simply a series of logistics potentially contributes to the marginalizing of her experiences as a pregnant woman, and specifically as a pregnant woman who in this case had previously given birth vaginally to her own children.

These types of marginalizing comments are amplified in the following three extracts, all from the same author. This author spent a considerable amount of time in his chapter on pregnancy writing negatively about the woman who carried his child, a woman who, like the woman in the previous extract, was also married and had children of her own. In the first extract from this author the woman who acted as the surrogate – Michelle – is depicted as mercenary, and as making poor decisions:

> Michelle has been doing a lot of complaining about money lately. First it was the compensation checks, now it's that her maternity allowance check is late. I keep wondering if it would be different if she had kept her job … She's also been talking a lot about how they've been spending the compensation money and I am feeling strange about that.
>
> *(Menichiello, 2012, n.p.)*

It is important to note that this was a compensated surrogacy arrangement organized through a clinic, involving a contract and a schedule of payments. To depict

Michelle as 'complaining about money' is, in effect, to ignore the inherently fiscal nature of the arrangement: it is only Michelle who is depicted as mercenary, rather than depicting all parties as potentially mercenary. The author then implicitly dismisses Michelle's 'complaints about money' by inferring that, had she kept her job, she wouldn't have money troubles. Despite having previously depicted Michelle as 'complaining about money', the author then goes on to act as though Michelle no longer has a job, thus dismissing her role as a surrogate as not a job (and hence outside the boundaries of all parties having rights and obligations). He then further emphasizes his concerns about Michelle by talking about how she has been spending money received as part of the contract. Indeed, a paragraph is later devoted to outlining what Michelle had spent money on, with items such as holidays implicitly depicted as a waste of money.

Whilst in extracts such as these the financial side of surrogacy arrangements was emphasized, in other instances the love side of surrogacy was emphasized, yet again in ways that potentially served to marginalize the experiences of women who act as surrogates. As the next extract from the same author again demonstrates – this time when reporting on a conversation with his partner – an emphasis upon altruism as a desirable characteristic of women who act as surrogates potentially serves to allow some gay men to claim that such women who should submit to the needs of gay men, rather than vice versa:

> 'It has been hard, I know. It's almost as though we're married to Michelle and James [Michelle's husband], isn't it' I asked. 'Whatever they do, whatever decision that they make directly affects us, and it's a feeling I can't get used to.'
>
> *(Menichiello, 2012, n.p.)*

This analogy to marriage mirrors analogies made by gay men in our research (Scholz & Riggs, 2014) on the topic of gay men who donate sperm to lesbian recipients. This research found that such men heterosexualize their relationship to lesbian recipients in order to claim a right to decision-making about children conceived of their donations. Whilst the analogy in the case of surrogacy doesn't per se heterosexualize the relationship between the gay men and the woman carrying a child for them (and her husband), it does remove the relationship from the realms of commercial surrogacy, instead locating it in the realm of the familial. Yet this appears to only work one way: the men are depicted as problematically impacted by the woman and her husband, yet the woman and her husband are not in turn seen as impacted by the gay men. The source of tension, then, is again the woman, not the surrogacy arrangement itself and the men's desire for it. In the third extract from this author below, the depiction of women who act as surrogates as a troubling imposition is most clearly stated:

> Our first thought was that there was no way that we could let Michelle pack up and move to Arizona being eight months pregnant with our child. It was

> way too risky. I put a call in to the same attorney who had been helping us with our prebirth order. 'I wouldn't let her move,' our attorney said. 'She's doing something wonderful for you, yes, that's a given, but there comes a time when you just have to put your foot down and say no, you're not moving.'
>
> *(Menichiello, 2012, n.p.)*

Prior to this extract the author had spent several pages discussing his anger at the fact that Michelle was moving to another state. In this extract both he and his male attorney are reported as sharing the view that, despite the contract not including terms preventing Michelle moving, the author should insist upon it. This was despite awareness that the move was important for Michelle and her family. This belief that intended parents should have the right to determine the movements of women who act as surrogates explicitly reduces such women to the role of service providers who, upon entering a contract to undertake a surrogacy arrangement, relinquish rights to their own autonomy. Whilst this was the most extreme example of such a belief, it was also evident in other books where a placenta previa meant that the woman was restricted to bed rest.

In the final extract below, the author who had negotiated with a friend to act as a surrogate comments on how the friendship was an imposition upon his experience of the pregnancy:

> Being friends with the surrogate has its advantages in so many ways, but it also definitely comes with its challenges. I wanted the pregnancy to be a beautiful experience. I wanted to cherish each step and each moment. However, it was very difficult to enjoy it when Mary was always feeling sick and exhausted. This affected her in many ways, not to mention her being hormonal because of being pregnant, and trying to be there for her was exhausting. I felt guilty and responsible and, at times, thought, *It would be so much easier if the surrogate just lived somewhere else and I wasn't having to go through all of this with her.* Being my surrogate's friend was often difficult for me.
>
> *(Warner, 2013, p. 41, original emphasis)*

In this extract, whilst the author acknowledges the positives of a surrogacy arrangement undertaken in the context of a friendship, his primary emphasis is on the negatives of such an arrangement. Specifically, whilst he reports empathy for the effects of the pregnancy upon Mary, his concern appears to lie primarily with the difficulties the friendship presented to him. Arguably, what is implied is that undertaking a surrogacy with someone he did not know would have allowed him to care less about the woman, and to instead focus on his own feelings. Again, such a desire depicts women who act as surrogates as an imposition on men who commission surrogacy arrangements.

Whilst it is important to acknowledge the often-complex journeys that some people undertake to become parents through surrogacy, the extracts included in this section highlight that it is also necessary to be aware of the ways in which some intending parents' desires and beliefs may lead to the reduction of women who act as surrogates to paid employees who must submit to the will of their employer. Whilst this may not be the intention of the parents analysed here, it is certainly a potential consequence of some of the ways in which they talk about the women who had acted as surrogates for them. As such, whilst the binary of love or money was apparent in the books we examined – much as it was apparent in the advertisements we considered in the previous section – ultimately it would appear that money constitutes an overriding framework that leads to beliefs about surrogacy amongst some intending parents where the role or contribution of the woman acting as a surrogate is minimized or marginalized. As we shall see in the following and final analytic section of this chapter, such minimizing is most clearly evident in accounts where intending parents claim the pregnancy as their own.

Claiming the pregnancy

Across the five books written by intending parents, the notion of a pregnancy being shared by the parents was a common trope, and one that was never problematized or questioned by the authors. Examples within the books include: 'Could it be that we were pregnant on our first attempt?' (Westoby, 2013, n.p.), 'Today marks the 35th day of our pregnancy … we have completed our seventh week of pregnancy' (Hirschi, 2014, n.p.) and 'The holidays were just around the corner. We also just entered our second trimester' (Warner, 2013, p. 43).

When examined in the abstract, it is possible to view these types of comments as the authors staking a claim to their child, a claim that arguably is important in regard to their future relationship with the child. At the same time, however, these comments typically appeared with sole reference to the couple. In other words, whilst it is not uncommon for a heterosexual cisgender couple where the female partner is pregnant for both the man and woman to claim that 'we're pregnant', in the examples provided above the claims were made solely about the intending parents, thus in effect excluding the woman who was actually pregnant.

The use of particular pronouns (i.e. 'we're pregnant') to stake a claim to the pregnancy was not the only way in which the authors did this. Some intending parents also made possessive claims about the woman who was carrying their child, such as: 'You really have to put a huge amount of trust in your surrogate' (Westoby, 2013, n.p.). This example demonstrates how particular descriptions of pregnant women in the context of surrogacy arrangements reduce such women to being the property of intended parents: 'your surrogate'. Another example of the reduction of women to their role in carrying a child appears as: 'Thing is, when our child is growing inside a womb 10,000 kilometres away, it's hard to wrap around the concept' (Hirschi, 2014, n.p.). In this example a pregnant woman in a surrogacy arrangement becomes just 'a womb', mirroring our concern earlier in this chapter about advertisements where women are reduced to 'carriers'.

Some intending parents also made claims to the pregnancy by naturalizing the entire surrogacy process as no different to a pregnancy undertaken by a woman who will be the mother to the child. This was most evident in the one book written by a heterosexual couple, as can be seen in the following quote: 'As Niall and I saw it, the development of our baby was just the same as a baby conceived in the normal way, only the insertion was different. Our baby wasn't a product but a living human being' (O'Flaherty & O'Flaherty, 2012). Here the female partner naturalizes a pregnancy through surrogacy as 'just the same as' a child conceived through reproductive heterosex, the only difference being the mode of 'insertion' (i.e. the implantation of the embryo). Not only does this form of strategic naturalization overlook the considerable degree of medical intervention involved in a surrogacy arrangement, but it also, we would suggest, allows for the implication that the pregnancy was that of the intending mother, not the woman carrying the child. If the development of the baby was 'just the same' (with the one difference being the mode of insertion), then 'just the same' means that the woman who will be the mother carries the child. Nowhere in this account is the role of the woman carrying the child spoken of. Whilst it might be suggested that these claims are a prelude to the final sentence, and are aimed at mitigating claims that surrogacy is a transactional arrangement involving the production of children, we would claim the opposite, namely that minimizing the role of the woman carrying the child highlights exactly how a logic of production (in which the 'manufacturer' of the 'goods' is removed from the equation) informs the statement made by these parents.

In sum, in this section we have provided examples of how, having first advertised for a surrogacy arrangement utilizing the language of both love and money, and then having apportioned love primarily to intending parents and issues over money primarily to women who act as surrogates, in the final analysis these both enable intending parents to then claim the pregnancy as their own. As we suggested in Chapter 1, the language of intent (here rendered within the guise of love) allows for the intending parents to be positioned as the only true stakeholders in the surrogacy arrangement: two make one.

Concluding thoughts

In this chapter we have emphasized how intending parents – enacting the role of agentic reproprenеurs – negotiate the binary of love and money, and in so doing demonstrate Zelizer's (2005) point that this binary is illusory. Specifically, our analysis of advertisements placed by intending parents and books written by such parents suggests that whilst the payment of money positions intending parents as authorizing the surrogacy arrangement, once this authorization has occurred (and their intent asserted), the language of payment is marginalized in favour of a narrative of love and desire. Women who act as surrogates, by contrast, are depicted as initially entering into the arrangements out of love (i.e. to help, or to give a gift), but once having entered into the arrangement they are then expected to act as though they are employees who must capitulate to the needs of their employer. The ultimate example of this appears in the capitulation to a narrative in which the pregnancy is attributed to the intending parents. Whilst, as we outlined earlier in this chapter, some women who act as surrogates refuse to capitulate (e.g. see Pande, 2009), the demand to accede to the intending parents is strong.

To return to our arguments in Chapter 1, we would suggest that the reversals of love and money outlined above serve to shift vulnerability from intending parents to women who act as surrogates. Advertising and paying for a surrogacy arrangement potentially signals a vulnerability, and certainly in some of the examples we have included in this chapter the vulnerability of intending parents (i.e. with regard to fertility) is explicitly commented on. Vulnerability, however, is replaced with agency as the intending parents successfully negotiate the marketplace, before ultimately laying claim to the pregnancy. Thus whilst, as Marilyn Strathern (1992) suggests, 'new techniques of "fertilisation" do not remedy fertility as such, but childlessness; they enable a potential parent to have access to the fertility of others' (p. 37), some intending parents appear to act as though their fertility concerns have indeed been remedied, allowing them to achieve a pregnancy. Elsewhere (Riggs & Due, 2013) we have expressed considerable concern about how this agentic narrative ignores the fact that parenting in general is often difficult, and that narratives of achievement and success as they frame surrogacy arrangements for many intending parents may do them a disservice in terms of being prepared for the journey that lies ahead. We have also expressed concern elsewhere (Riggs & Due, 2010) that attempts at minimizing the vulnerability of intending parents potentially leads to a lack of awareness or insight into the potential vulnerabilities then produced for women who act as surrogates (as we explored in the previous chapter).

In contrast to our suggestion in Chapter 1, then, that an orientation to surrogacy must involve a turning to the face of the Other, it would appear, at least from our analysis presented in this chapter, that if anything surrogacy produces in intending parents a turning *away* from the face of the Other. A turning away both from the vulnerability of the self, and also a turning away from how we are constituted through our relationships with others. In many ways, it would appear, the very fact of the Other is relegated to the margins in the accounts of intending parents. This is an issue we will take up in greater detail in the final chapter of this book, where we explore how capitalism potentially produces this orientation away from the face of the Other, and how alternate modes of becoming orientated might be possible.

What also disappears in the accounts we have examined in this chapter is the extent to which pronatalism informs the accounts. The desire not simply to parent a child, but to parent a genetically related child, only serves to reinforce the privilege accorded to such parent–child relations, and to reinforce the idea that reproduction is inherently good for the planet and all who live on it. The narrative of conquest and mastery inherent to surrogacy arrangements thus only serves to reinforce a pronatalist logic, and more broadly to reinforce a capitalist system of exchange where the services of others can be bought so as to allow certain adults a place within the realms of reproductive citizenship. These are concerns that we take up in further detail in the following chapter, when we turn to examine how children born through surrogacy arrangements are understood and represented.

5

CHILDREN AND SURROGACY

Overview

In Chapter 2 we argued that in capitalist societies children are increasingly seen as priceless and precious, yet at the same time their value is not outside of a capitalist logic. Whilst this might seem counterintuitive (i.e. that a child could be priceless and yet have a value), we argued in Chapter 2 that the increasing emphasis placed upon genetic relatedness has meant that certain children are perhaps valued more than others. As a result, whilst the norm of reproductive citizenship privileges those who have children over those who do not, it would appear to us that particular modes of having children result in kinship relations that are seen as more valued than others. It is in this sense that all children are seen as priceless, yet some as potentially more valuable.

In this chapter we consider how these messages of pricelessness and value appear in storybooks written for children conceived and born through surrogacy arrangements. Specifically, we focus on six such books: *The Very Kind Koala* (Kluger-Bell, 2013), *Why I'm So Special: A Book About Surrogacy* (Lewis-Long, 2010), *Why I'm So Special: A Book About Surrogacy with Two Daddies* (Lewis-Long, 2011), *Sophia's Broken Crayons* (Falk, 2014), *The Kangaroo Pouch* (Phillips Pellet, 2006) and *Will and Hope have a Baby: The Gift of Surrogacy* (Celcer, 2014). In examining these books we consider the messages they contain with regard to intending parents (specifically in relation to how the books naturalize the injunction to have children), women who act as surrogates (specifically how the books take up the discourses we explored in Chapter 3 with regard to altruism) and how they depict children born of surrogacy arrangements as priceless.

We are very aware, in a book that seeks to represent all parties involved in surrogacy arrangements, that our use of storybooks does not necessarily represent the views of children. In identifying the data that we would examine in this chapter we were faced with limitations currently inherent to the study of surrogacy, namely that very little research (as we shall see below) has included the voices of children. Indeed, to date our own research has not involved speaking with children conceived through surrogacy arrangements. Whilst it might be argued that this is a product of the fact that commercial surrogacy arrangements have dramatically increased only over the past decade (and so the children are still young), Ragoné's work on surrogacy arrangements is now over two decades old, and the children born to the intending parents interviewed for her book would now be adults. It is thus notable that researchers to date have not engaged substantively with these adults, nor indeed that the adults themselves do not appear to have written publicly about their experiences. In regard to other possible accounts of children, the majority of media reports that have included a substantive focus on children have, unfortunately, been negative (specifically with regard to recent cases where children have allegedly been abandoned by intending parents, as we will discuss briefly below).

In focusing on children's storybooks, then, we are mindful of the limitations of this approach, but nonetheless suggest that such a focus is useful for two reasons. First, it is likely that the storybooks have been, and will continue to be, read to young children. As such, the narratives within the books we examine will potentially make a formative contribution to how children who read them understand surrogacy arrangements. Second, the narratives contained within the books – like narratives in all storybooks – arguably demonstrate what adult authors believe will be intelligible to young children. Focusing on how surrogacy is made intelligible to child readers is thus a potentially important undertaking when it comes to understanding how children as potential future research participants may frame their experiences, in addition to highlighting what children born through surrogacy arrangements potentially represent to their parents. Before presenting our analysis of the narratives contained in the books, we first examine the limited previous research on children conceived and born through surrogacy arrangements, focusing specifically on:

1 cases where children have allegedly been abandoned;
2 accounts provided by intending parents with regard to how they explain surrogacy to their children; and
3 research on outcomes for children, including the one study that has reported children's voices.

The lives of children born through surrogacy arrangements

Given our claim that children are increasingly seen as priceless, it is perhaps atypical that recent high-profile cases have been reported in which intending parents have allegedly abandoned a child or children born for them. Yet this can be explained following an argument that we have elaborated in detail elsewhere (Riggs & Peel, 2016), namely that whilst as a general principle children may be valued, such valuation is premised upon conformity to a particular set of norms. Not only are children who are genetically related to their parents particularly valued, but so too are children who are neurotypical or who do not otherwise fall within categories that may be labelled as exhibiting a disability. This is not to say that parents of children living with disabilities do not love their children. Rather, it is to suggest that the idealization of children brings with it the image of a particular form of idealized child. When children are born who do not conform to an idealized image, some parents frame this as a loss. Whilst the abandonment of a child is an extreme response to such experiences of loss, we would argue that it is part of a broader logic in which certain children are culturally valued more than others, and that the devaluation of certain children can lead parents to particular extreme responses.

In the context of surrogacy, one particular surrogacy arrangement has received considerable media attention, namely the case of Baby Gammy. As Brianne Richards (2015) argues, given the lengths that intending parents often go to in order to have a child through a surrogacy arrangement, it may seem surprising that cases of abandonment occur. Yet as Richards notes, 'unfortunately … incidents of child abandonment are not isolated' (p. 203). In the case of Baby Gammy, an Australian heterosexual couple commissioned a surrogacy arrangement in Thailand. Late in the pregnancy it was identified that one of the two children being carried as part of this arrangement had Down syndrome, and the intending parents indicated that they wished for the child to be aborted. The woman carrying the children refused this, as it contravened her religious beliefs. When the children were born, the intended parents travelled to Thailand but only returned to Australia with the child who did not have Down syndrome. At the time it was reported in the media that the children's father had stated that '[t]here is a normal one, can I take the normal one?' (Richards, 2015, p. 212). However, more recently the Western Australian Family Court has found that the intended parents did not abandon one of their children, instead suggesting that one of the children remained in Thailand because the woman who carried the children refused to relinquish one of them (ABC News, 2016). Whatever the facts of the matter were (and it does not surprise us that the latest turn of events with regards to the case has involved blaming the woman who carried the children), as Richards notes, the alleged abandonment of children born through surrogacy arrangements does occur – even if it is limited to a small number of cases. Again, whilst children in general are increasingly seen as valuable and precious, it is nonetheless the case that some children are valued more than others, as the Baby Gammy case would seem to indicate.

Whilst narratives of abandonment have dominated the media to a certain degree in recent years with regards to surrogacy, they are a world away from the narratives that intending parents in general voice about surrogacy. Common within the narratives of such parents are metaphors used to describe why surrogacy was necessary. In her early research in the field Ragoné (1994) reported that many of the intending parents she interviewed in the United States utilized the narrative of having a 'broken tummy' in order to legitimize surrogacy (p. 134). Two decades later, and the same narratives are evident in UK research: 'Mummy's tummy was broken and [surrogate] offered to help us and so the doctors gave daddy some special equipment and he put his seeds in there and then [surrogate] put the seeds inside her so you could grow' (Blake, Zadeh, Statham & Freeman, 2014, p. 258).

These types of narratives repeat the claims we made in Chapter 4, namely that narratives of surrogacy amongst intending parents typically involve a shift from a narrative of loss associated with infertility, to one involving agency. Yet echoing to a degree our arguments in Chapters 1 and 2, the shift from vulnerability to agency typically involves the instrumentalization of women who act as surrogates. A consistent example of this across the literature appears in the metaphor of the surrogate womb as an 'oven'. Jennifer Readings and her colleagues (2011) note that one of their participants had explained surrogacy to their child as 'We've made it like a bread in the oven, she just kept you warm until you were ready to come out' (p. 491). Murphy (2015) similarly reports that one of the gay intending parents he interviewed planned to tell his children that 'she carried them like in an oven until they were ready and then she gave them to us' (p. 187). So dominant is this narrative, it would appear, that women who act as surrogates have been reported as taking up this narrative, as noted by Jacobson (2016), who reports that one of the women she interviewed described herself as 'just an oven' (p. 57).

In these narratives of surrogacy as akin to baking 'bread in the oven', it could be suggested that not only are women's bodies instrumentalized, but so too are children. If women are reduced to mere ovens (which naturalizes women's reproductive capacity through the analogy to ovens, whose sole purpose it is to bake things), then the analogy of children to baked bread similarly reduces children as goods produced for consumption. The difference between the two we would argue, however, is that whilst women who act as surrogates are reduced to objects of production, children are positioned as desirable goods that are produced. The journey from the 'broken tummy' to the child 'baked in the oven' is thus a journey from vulnerability to agency on the part of intending parents, just as it is a journey from desiring to having the object of one's desire.

This journey from reproductive vulnerability to having the object of one's desire is drawn upon in the research of Susan Golombok and her colleagues (2004) to account for their finding that their participants who had children through surrogacy provided more positive accounts of parenting than did their participants who had children through reproductive heterosex. Given the cost and stress of surrogacy arrangements, in addition to the potential distress caused by infertility, they suggest 'it is not surprising, therefore, that those who do become parents at the end of this difficult process are highly involved with their much-wanted children' (p. 408). Importantly, however, Golombok and her colleagues note that participants who had their children through surrogacy arrangements were 'emotionally overinvolved' with their children when compared with participants who had their children through reproductive heterosex, though they note that the degree of overinvolvement was not at a 'pathological level' (p. 409). It is unsurprising to us, given the discourse of children as priceless, that those who go to the greatest lengths to have children would report the greatest investment, given their journey to becoming parents has been explicitly framed by investments all along.

Turning to consider the one study that has reported on children's voices, Vasanti Jadva and her colleagues (2012) report that some of their young participants drew upon similar narratives to those outlined above. For example, one young person noted 'Well my Mum's womb, I think … well it was a bit broken, so … [surrogate] carried me instead of Mum' (p. 3011). Their views of the women who carried them were also elicited, with one young participant describing the woman who carried them as 'kind and she's lovely and funny' (p. 3011). Turning to consider surrogacy arrangements in general, one child appeared to engage in the kind of strategic naturalization we discussed in Chapter 1, stating that 'It's just pretty much nature so I can't do anything about it' (p. 3012). Children such as this appeared pragmatic in their accounts of surrogacy, accepting it as a necessity for their own birth, whilst also seemingly being aware that their birth needed to be framed as 'pretty much nature' so as to legitimate the arrangement itself.

As we noted above, the literature on children in the context of surrogacy is relatively limited. Of course it could be suggested that *all* of the literature on surrogacy is about children, given it involves research about the process of having children. Our interest in this section, however, has been to focus on how children themselves are accounted for. It would appear to us that many of the narratives both about and by children draw upon the wider tropes that circulate with regard to the topic of surrogacy, and which either implicitly or explicitly frame surrogacy as a mode of labour, a mode of production, and thus engage with the logic of capitalism. Whilst to a certain degree there is a disorientation at play in the metaphors that are used (such as can be seen in the quote from the young person who referred to surrogacy as 'pretty much nature'), such disorientation is arguably produced by the norm of reproductive heterosex, in which the creation of children outside of this norm produces a vulnerability. Yet as we shall see in our analysis of the six storybooks, and much as we have argued throughout this book, disorientation is ultimately triumphed by claims to agency and a subsequent reinsertion of intending parents and their children into normative kinship narratives.

Storybook analysis

In our examination of the six storybooks, we identified six common tropes across the books that, when combined, serve to produce a relatively homogenous account of surrogacy arrangements. The first of these tropes evoked the idea that having children is part of a normative relationship life course. Elsewhere (Riggs & Bartholomaeus, 2016) we have suggested that the evocation of a normative relationship life course trajectory serves to naturalize reproduction by treating it as axiomatic, rather than as a culturally produced expectation. This point is perhaps especially salient in the context of surrogacy, where the 'natural' in reproduction (i.e. reproductive heterosex) is shown to be unachievable (i.e. due to medical or social infertility), and thus a surrogacy arrangement is required to 'supplement' the reproductivity of one or both partners in a couple.

Specifically in terms of having children as a normative part of adult relationships, in some of the books with human characters (e.g. Lewis-Long, 2010, 2011) a life course narrative was evoked in which the intending parents went through a journey from meeting, dating, marriage and then the expectation of children. Books with non-human characters (e.g. koalas, kangaroos) provided a narrative in which the intending parents saw other animals with babies, leading them too to want to have children (e.g. Kluger-Bell, 2013; Phillips Pellet, 2006). In examples such as these, two differing, though complementary, accounts of children as part of a normative relationship life course are provided. In the first, and in the books where the protagonists are either koalas or kangaroos, it is stated that the desire for a child is produced by a broader social context in which reproductivity is normalized. Importantly, however, this does not appear to be a critique of such normalization, but rather both of the books implicitly treat the fact that other people having children means that the protagonists should desire to have children too (i.e. rather than questioning whether they want children at all). Whilst it could be argued that representations of the cultural context in which the desire for children becomes intelligible draw attention to the culturally produced injunction to have children, it is unlikely that this message would be intelligible to young readers.

The second way in which children are treated as a normative part of adult relationships is in the suggestion that the parents had 'naturally' gotten to a stage in their relationship where children were the logical next step. As we suggested in Chapter 4, accounts such as these valorize families with children as the only true families, thus creating a paired contrast with families that do not involve children, and who are by implication located outside of the category 'family'. With these points in mind about the injunction to have children and the apportioning of the category 'family' only to families that have children, we can see that these books from the onset position children as priceless and desirable.

The second trope in the books echoes our summary of the previous literature above, namely in the use of the 'broken tummy' narrative. Given our points above about the injunction to, and naturalization of, reproductivity, it is perhaps understandable that the books are required to produce an argument as to why the parents have, in effect, failed to fulfil roles that are treated as natural, yet why they then persist in the face of this failure. Examples from the books include reference to women with broken bellies, an inability to carry a child, and as something otherwise being wrong with the woman's uterus (e.g. Celcer, 2014; Falk, 2014; Kluger-Bell, 2013; Lewis-Long, 2010, 2011). Whilst these accounts emphasize women's purported reproductive failures, the inclusion of a book featuring gay fathers (Lewis-Long, 2011) in the sample of storybooks is useful, as it highlights how the injunction to reproductivity is differentially distributed according to gender. In all of the books besides the one featuring two men, it is women's bodies that are depicted as failing what is otherwise treated as their natural role: to reproduce. Whilst this failure is localized to particular body parts, these body parts are always connected to women through the possessive noun that proceeds them. As synecdoches for the women themselves, then, the failure is not limited to particular body parts, but by implication is generalized to the women themselves. Men, by contrast, are not accorded the same status as having failed, given the dominant cultural assumption that men are not made for carrying children. Whilst this ignores the fact that some transgender men might indeed carry babies, within this sample of storybooks men are exempt from narratives of failure because they are exempt from the demand to gestation.

As we have argued in other chapters, however, this depiction of failure is quickly replaced by a narrative of agency, in the form of a third trope evident in the storybooks in which intending parents identify alternate ways of having a child. Many examples of this include the intending parents actively seeking out a doctor for help, a doctor that they can easily access, who knows how to help them, and who provides a quick and easy solution to their problem (e.g. Celcer, 2014; Kluger-Bell, 2013; Lewis-Long, 2010). Importantly, these doctors do not appear in the books out of nowhere. Rather, the intending parents actively seek them out, both relying on the doctors' knowledge of surrogacy, but also knowing that their own agency is necessary in order to provide redress for their infertility.

Importantly, whilst the intending parents are often depicted as presenting to the doctor with sadness, this sadness very quickly turns to joy, which is depicted as a product of their agency. Our point here is not to suggest that intending parents should always be sad, or should remain sad. Rather, our point is how agency directed towards having children becomes the naturalized response to infertility (as opposed to, for example, deciding not to have children). Further, our concern, and one we have explored in detail elsewhere (Riggs, 2015b), is with how the desire to have a child leads intending parents to surrogacy, rather than other pathways such as foster care or adoption. All six books treat as axiomatic that if a woman (or gay couple) cannot carry a child, then they will find someone else to carry a child for them. Excluded from this, then, are alternate possible pathways to parenthood.

Once surrogacy is established as the only (and indeed automatic) option for intending parents who cannot carry a child, all of the books then draw upon a fourth trope, namely the construction of women who act as surrogates as willing, and indeed joyous, parties to the arrangement. In such representations women who act as surrogates are depicted as happy and as enjoying their role, as naturally fulfilling their capacity as women (i.e. able to carry children), and often as nice and caring (e.g. Celcer, 2014; Kluger-Bell, 2013; Lewis-Long, 2010, 2011). Across this gamut of positive affirmations, however, is one key word that, we would suggest, unite these affirmations into one coherent category: helpful. Dayna Evans (2015) has argued that the language of 'helping' is specifically gendered, typically only applied to women. In the context of surrogacy a woman who 'helps', we would argue, is reduced to a supplementary role that is treated as entirely axiomatic with what is expected of her as a woman. In other words, not only is she helping someone do something that is implicitly depicted as natural (i.e. the desire to have a child), but her helping is treated as a natural by-product of the fact that she can reproduce.

For us the language of 'helping' echoes Strathern's (2003) concerns about the ways in which the language of 'assisted reproduction' naturalizes all forms of reproduction, and Roach Anleu's (1992) concern about the ways in which narratives of surrogacy naturalize women's labour in the context of surrogacy arrangements. To 'help' someone have a child by carrying a child for them becomes a normative expectation of women, one devoid in the books of the possible negative implications of pregnancy and childbirth (including possible miscarriages, difficulties in birthing the child, and the potential distress that may be associated with relinquishing the child after they are born).

Paired with the naturalization of women's 'helping' role is a fifth trope, involving the assertion within the storybooks that it is the intent of the parents that determines whose contribution to the creation of the child counts the most. This primarily occurred through reference to babies born going 'back' to their intending parents. In her interviews with women who have acted as surrogates, Jacobson (2016) suggests that such women often use the language of 'giving babies back rather than giving babies up' (p. 58). This type of narrative, Jacobson suggests, serves to mitigate any distress that women may face in relinquishing a child they have carried once they are born. We would suggest further that the language of 'giving back' serves to insist, as we argued in Chapter 1, that it is the intent of the parents that constitutes the strongest claim to the child. The language of giving back, however, ignores the fact that the intending parents did not hand over a child to be cared for, to then have that child handed back to them. Rather, what the woman who carries the child receives is either an embryo (in the case of gestational surrogacy) or genetic material (in the case of traditional surrogacy). Treating the genetic materials of the intending parents as a child before implantation accords to them a determining role in the creation of the child, and thus to a certain degree discounts the role of the woman who carries the child.

Understandably, all of the books conclude with a sixth trope, namely the birth of the child. Yet the books go beyond simply celebrating the birth, and instead evoke language that signifies the pricelessness of the child themselves. For example, children are referred to as special, and as a gift (Celcer, 2014; Falk, 2014; Lewis-Long, 2011). Echoing our arguments in Chapter 2, children born of surrogacy arrangements are priceless, 'special' 'gifts' given to intending parents. It is interesting to us that the language of 'gifts' is evoked in the books. As Teman (2010) notes, the language of gift-giving in the context of surrogacy is vexed, as typically a gift relationship evokes reciprocity, yet it is questionable as to what women who act as surrogates receive in return. One answer to this question is provided above, in the paired framing of women 'helping' intending parents and then 'giving back' a child. If women's helping role is naturalized, and the child is positioned as always already belonging to the intending parents, then there is no reciprocity required: to help is not to expect reciprocity, and to return something to its rightful owner does not necessarily bring with it an expectation of reciprocity.

Interestingly, in the book that featured two men, the act of giving something back to the woman who carried the child is explicitly mentioned, but only in this one book. In this book, the intending parents take the woman who will carry their child on an overseas holiday and buy her a dog. Given the author of this book has written a similar book on a heterosexual couple entering into a surrogacy arrangement (Lewis-Long, 2010), and that in this book no mention is made of gifts to the woman who carries the child, it is notable to us that commerce is only a feature of the one book featuring a gay couple. We might conjecture that this reflects wider cultural narratives about heterosexual as compared to gay couples entering into surrogacy arrangements. In our interviews with Australian heterosexual intending parents, a number suggested that their journey was different to gay men, because gay men did not have to cope with the distress of medical infertility (see also Lewin, 2009). We might suggest that the storybooks similarly frame heterosexual couples as having troubling journeys from infertility to agency, and that the 'helping' provided to them by women who carry children for them becomes a naturalized response to another's distress. For gay men in comparison, perhaps, there is an implicit assertion of 'choice' on the part of gay men to have a child, a choice that then brings with it a demand for reciprocity (Lewin, 2009). Certainly in our other work we have demonstrated that gay men are depicted as engaging in a 'lifestyle choice' when entering into surrogacy arrangements, and that such a 'choice' is not inherently deserving of support (Collins, Riggs & Due, 2014). That gay men who make this 'choice' should solely be depicted within the books as needing to reciprocate thus perhaps reflects broader cultural narratives about which intending parents are more deserving than others.

To return to the final trope, that of the priceless child, it would thus appear that within the storybooks children are indeed depicted as priceless, and that this claim is bolstered through the idea that, in all of the books bar one, there is no reciprocity required from intending parents to the women who carry their children. This suggests to us that whilst children may be priceless (at least in the context of heterosexual relationships), women are very specifically valued for the 'help' they can provide. Implicit to this, then, is the message to young readers that whilst they may be priceless, the same may not necessarily be true for the women who carried and birthed them. Whilst there is certainly a value attached to women who act as surrogates within the books, this value would appear to be time-limited, yet at the same time the value associated with the labour engaged in by women is located outside of a logic of reciprocity. As we have argued in Chapters 1 and 2, this is a very particular logic of capitalism, one in which the producer of a good can be alienated from the goods that they produce, and further that being capable of producing a particular good does not automatically entitle one to reciprocity. Whilst these meanings we have imputed to the storybooks are likely far beyond the intentions of their authors, they serve to highlight the potential messages that they provide to young readers.

Concluding thoughts

As we noted in the introduction to this chapter, it is arguably the case that children are always the focus when we consider the ways in which we orientate ourselves to the topic of surrogacy. Were it not for the value accorded to reproductivity, and the privileging of families that involve children, the instrumentalization that underpins surrogacy arrangements might not be intelligible. Yet in becoming orientated to the topic of surrogacy, it is easy to focus solely upon either the instrumentalization of women who act as surrogates, or the decisions and motivations of people who enter into surrogacy arrangements. Missing from this story is an orientation to how children conceived and born through surrogacy arrangements are understood. In this chapter we have attempted to make a contribution to the small body of literature that focuses on such children. Our contribution is limited by our focus on children's storybooks, yet we would repeat our earlier claim that these books are of interest both for how they display what adults think should be intelligible to children, and potentially for the messages that young readers may take from the books, including about their parents, the women who carried them, and of course themselves.

With regard to our argument about the conflict between priceless children and the value attached to children, in this chapter we have demonstrated how this pairing functions (at least within the storybooks we examined), by emphasizing how surrogacy is treated as a default option for couples who cannot bear a child themselves. Ignored in these accounts are other ways of having children, or indeed not having children at all (and thus reinforcing the human exceptionalism that we have suggested sits at the heart of surrogacy arrangements, and indeed the injunction to reproductivity more broadly). Echoing our points in Chapter 2, then, the books appear to mirror the historical and cultural shift away from *any* child being a priceless object, to only particular children being especially valued. Whilst the books do not substantively engage with the topic of genetics (though certainly *Will and Hope have a Baby* (Celcer, 2014) does discuss eggs and sperm and their role in the creation of a child), they nonetheless treat as taken-for-granted that parents will create a child 'of their own', rather than raise a child created by someone else who is then unable to raise the child. As books written to support families formed through surrogacy, it is of course understandable that the books would valorize surrogacy. Yet it is important for us to question at what expense, and how this further endorses the norm of genetic relatedness in which only certain children are seen as priceless.

Also evident in the storybooks is a familiar trope that we have already explored in this book, namely how vulnerability is replaced by agency. In all of the books the intending parents shift from despair to hope, from lack to fulfilment. Yet whilst women who act as surrogates are very much part of the story, we would not go so far as to suggest that this represents a turn towards the face of the Other with regard to vulnerability. Doing so would involve recognizing how the Other too despairs and lacks, just as how the Other hopes and is fulfilled. It could be suggested that the female characters who act as surrogates are accorded happiness in being able to 'help', and certainly in the book featuring the gay couple it could be suggested that the woman is lacking (given they need to buy things for her). But this is not the same as truly considering the material and emotional contexts in which women who act as surrogates live.

Turning to face the Other, then, in the context of the storybooks is more like a glance towards another before turning back to the self. There is no double turn as Ahmed (2004) suggests is needed, there is no acknowledgement of the differential distribution of vulnerability, and there is no sustained acknowledged of the fact of the Other as a foundation of the self. Of course it could be argued that these are children's storybooks, and none of this could be achieved in such a context. We would suggest, by contrast, that it is the orientation towards surrogacy that the books adopt that is the problem, not the requirements of child readers. In other words, it would be entirely possible for a storybook about surrogacy to clearly and critically situate the intending parents in broader cultural contexts, just as it would be entirely possible to talk more transparently about the journeys of women who act as surrogates. That the books do not do this signals their orientation towards surrogacy as a capitalist enterprise of production in which agency is privileged over vulnerability.

Finally, it is interesting to note that the storybooks we examined largely avoided the binary of love and money that was so salient in Chapters 3 and 4. Other than the book focused on two fathers, no mention is made in the books of payment to women who act as surrogates. In this sense, the children are indeed priceless. Yet this pricelessness is dependent on the naturalization of women's labour, where women who act as surrogates are depicted as 'helping' intending parents, thus reinforcing the idea that this is a role that women (albeit 'special', 'nice' women) should undertake simply because they can. Yet locating surrogacy outside of a market economy, as the books do, does not mean that a market economy does not operate within the books. Rather, the market itself is naturalized through gendered narratives that render invisible women's labour. Given that the research of Jadva and her colleagues (2012) suggests that children conceived through surrogacy are aware of the labour undertaken on their behalf, and indeed many such children wish to develop relationships with the women who carried them, it is to a certain degree disingenuous that the storybooks we examined in this chapter minimize the labour aspects of surrogacy, instead focusing solely or primarily on narratives of agency and assistance. As we shall see in the following chapter, clinics that facilitate surrogacy arrangements play a key role in perpetuating this invisibilization, and form another (potentially key) spoke in the wheel upon which the instrumentalization of women's bodies in the name of capital rests.

6

SURROGACY CLINICS

Overview

As we suggested in Chapter 4, many intending parents who commission surrogacy arrangements assert a claim to agency through adopting the role of represpreneur, actively engaging with the fertility market so as to achieve their desire to have a child. As the literature summarized more broadly in Chapters 1 and 2 would suggest, fertility markets promote a particular idealized vision of parenthood that is reliant upon the invisibilization of women's labour in the context of surrogacy, by and large reducing the bodies of women who act as surrogates to raw materials whose purpose is the production of goods. Indeed, it was interesting for us to learn that the etymology of the word 'material' is derived from the word 'mater', or mother. Whilst there are multiple ways in which this derivation can be construed, it is certainly the case that the word material (as substance, as object) is derived from the word mother. That we potentially see a new iteration of the reduction of women to materials in the context of surrogacy is of considerable interest to us throughout this book.

Bearing in mind our note above about the etymology of the word 'material', in this chapter we focus on how the websites of surrogacy clinics often appear to rely upon the taken-for-grantedness of women's bodies when marketing to intending parents. Specifically, we suggest that women's bodies are so naturalized within the websites of surrogacy clinics that they almost disappear. Whilst it is understandable that any business will primarily speak to potential customers (rather than to those who produce the goods they are selling), it would not be atypical for a business to also speak *about* the goods that they are selling and how they are made. In the case of surrogacy, however, speaking about women who act as surrogates as producers of goods does not align with the ways in which surrogacy services and the cultural contexts they exist within attempt to mitigate the commodification of women's bodies by focusing on narratives of choice and agency. It would appear, however, that rather than speaking directly about concerns over commodification, or even attempting to provide a narrative that sidesteps concerns about commodification, surrogacy clinic websites almost take it as a fait accompli that women's bodies are reduced to the material they can produce in the context of surrogacy.

In order to provide some substance to the claims made above, in this chapter we present an analysis of the information provided about surrogacy pathways available to gay men on twelve clinic websites. We decided to focus solely on websites that target gay men so as to limit the data set. There are a much larger number of websites that focus on heterosexual intending parents, and the information provided to such parents is much more extensive. Collating and analysing such a potentially large data set was beyond our focus and intentions for this chapter, especially given websites targeting heterosexual intending parents have already been examined (as we discuss below). Further, given our previous arguments about the naturalization of surrogacy as a proxy for reproductive heterosex, it seemed important to us to examine how gay men are invited to take up the injunction to reproduce. As our analysis demonstrates, advertising targeted at gay men suggests that very similar logics are employed by clinics regardless of the target audience, and that this is a product of a capitalist logic underpinning service provision.

In terms of the data, all of the websites were for clinics located in the Americas. Whilst at the time when we collected and analysed these data in late 2015 surrogacy was possible for gay men in Mexico, this situation has since changed. We have, however, opted to retain the twelve websites in our sample, given, as we shall see below, their relative homogeneity in terms of messages to intending parents. Focusing on gay intending parents as they are framed by the websites provides us an opportunity both to focus on the identities made available to gay men on the websites (as agentic repropreneurs), and the corresponding ways in which women who act as surrogates are depicted. Before presenting our analysis, however, we first outline previous research that has explored the ways in which surrogacy clinics advertise to intending parents.

Marketing surrogacy

In terms of previous research, Lauren Jade Martin (2015) focuses on surrogacy clinic websites in her book *Reproductive Tourism in the United States*. Martin makes a distinction between active marketing undertaken by surrogacy clinics (such as providing seminars aimed at marketing services to potential intending parents), and passive marketing, specifically websites. Martin (2015) suggests that websites may be especially useful for attracting potential clients transnationally:

> Although many providers claimed not to aggressively market their services abroad, their web presence functions at least as a passive form of marketing. According to my informants, their domestic and international clients find them via the Internet. Global fertility markets are dependent upon technology for the

> spread of information, enabling intended parents to virtually shop for global fertility services through Internet searches and the viewing of websites of clinics and programs.
>
> *(p. 97)*

To a certain degree, we would question the distinction between active and passive marketing, particularly given the globalization of surrogacy services. Bearing in mind that the pursuit of capital involves identifying the most cost-effective means of promoting one's services, it is arguably the case that travelling to countries where potential customers might live is not a cost-effective means of promoting one's service. In this sense, then, clinic websites might not be the 'passive form of marketing' that Martin and her interviewees suggest them to be. Indeed, Martin suggests as much when she goes on to state that:

> Promoting one's service with a website is particularly important for some programs that wish to reach a global audience, and some clinics and programs tailor their Internet presence to this market by translating their sites into multiple languages, or by having special pages specifically targeting people who may be coming from out of state or abroad … This kind of passive marketing is especially important in countries where physicians and lawyers are prohibited from advertising and soliciting in television or print media.
>
> *(2005, p. 97)*

Whilst in this quote Martin continues to use the language of 'passive marketing', we would locate this within the context of her suggestion that aiming to reach a 'global audience' in which certain countries may prohibit advertising in television or print media is a key agenda of surrogacy clinics. Developing a clearly branded website that is purposively indexed by search engines targeting key words likely to be used by intending parents as they 'do the research' is thus perhaps less passive than it is an intentional and active approach to targeting potential intending parents. Furthermore, as Murphy (2015) suggests in his consideration of promotional materials utilized by surrogacy clinics that target gay men: 'the advertising strategies and linguistic choices of commercial surrogacy agencies play a role in shaping th[e] desire [of gay men], particularly through promoting their services via information sessions, statements in the media, and on their own websites' (p. 108). We build upon this suggestion by Murphy in our analysis below, but suffice it to say here that whilst the desires of gay men to become parents are shaped by the cultural contexts in which they live – where reproductive citizenship is valorized and where a pronatalist logic is endorsed – they are then further validated by surrogacy clinics which draw upon culturally available narratives to shape their promotional materials in ways that are likely to be attractive to potential gay intending parents.

Part of the ways in which surrogacy clinic websites authorize the desire of gay men is to, from the onset, shape the roles of each of the parties involved in surrogacy arrangements. As we shall see in our analysis below, this involves depicting women who act as surrogates in very specific ways. Whilst little attention has been paid in previous research to how advertising materials depict women who act as surrogates, sustained attention has been paid to how surrogacy clinics more broadly mediate the relationships between intending parents and women who act as surrogates, and indeed how clinics mediate both intending parents' and women's relationships with themselves. Rudrappa and Collins (2015) outline this clearly with regard to surrogacy clinics in India:

> Surrogacy agencies actively control the images of the surrogate mothers that circulate in popular media, and among clients: First, the agencies *all* speak about how well they treat surrogate mothers, and how happy the women are to be of service to others. Second, surrogate mothers are characterized as generous yet desperately poor individuals who are good mothers. Third, they are also depicted as shy, sensitive, and secretive about their choice, eager to return back to their own families, and unwilling or unable to speak with clients, researchers, or journalists … Many surrogacy agencies maintain websites with pictures of smiling, pregnant surrogate mothers and infants. These websites feature information about why Indian women pursue surrogacy, the rigorous psychological and medical testing they undergo, and how their lives are improved by becoming a surrogate mother.
>
> *(pp. 10–11)*

As we suggested in the introduction to this chapter, and argue in the analysis below, the websites we examined did little in the way of providing the types of positive representations that Rudrappa and Collins suggest circulate within the context of Indian surrogacy clinics. Their final suggestion about how women who may potentially act as surrogates are screened, however, is certainly echoed in our findings below. The depiction of women who act as surrogates as clearly managed through screening processes is part of a wider narrative promoted by surrogacy clinics, in which both intending parents and women who act as surrogates are socialized into relationships that centre upon commerce, as Vora (2014) has suggested:

> Structures and practices in the clinic endeavor to separate social relationships from reproductive bodies, and the negotiation of this separation is one of the most evident efforts in the experimental social relations formed and imagined in the clinic … Though these relationships are not at the heart of the clinic's intended goals for surrogacy, they support its success … These experimental relations can be understood to reflect or react to, in part, an intentional shift in medicine and governmentality away from a technique of caring for the body, or pastoral care, to one of producing bodies as the instruments of service work and surrogates as entrepreneurs of the contracted use of those instruments.
>
> *(pp. 64–65)*

Vora's work is important for the ways in which accounts of the (often caring) relationships that may be engendered between intending parents and women who act as surrogates (as evident in previous research, such as by Ragoné, 1994, and Teman, 2010) are always already mediated by the instrumentalization of reproduction and its incorporation into a capitalist logic of production. As we shall now see in our analysis, this logic is clearly evident in surrogacy clinic websites, thus suggesting that intending parents may be inculcated into this logic from their very first point of contact with a potential service.

Surrogacy websites which target gay men

As we indicated in the introduction to this chapter, in examining the twelve websites we only focus on information pertaining to gay intending parents. Specifically, we focused on how gay men are interpellated as repropreneurs within the advertising materials on the websites, and in so doing we identified three key ways that the websites hail gay men as parents-to-be. Having presented these below, we then turn to focus on how women who act as surrogates are depicted. Echoing our claims in the introduction to this chapter, on many of the websites women who act as surrogates were all but invisible. When they were visible, as we shall see, they were depicted in ways that were highly regulatory and instrumentalized.

'Having it your way': the neoliberal consumer

The title of this first mode of address directed at potential gay intending parents comes from the *Growing Generations* website. The opening phrase on the page that specifically speaks to gay men is 'Having it your way'. These words encapsulate the neoliberal framing of commercial surrogacy for gay men across many of the websites. Specifically, the phrase frames gay men's desire to become parents as something that should rightfully be tailored to gay men's lives. This idea of surrogacy services being targeted to suit gay men was evident on two other websites:

> Our expert level of care goes beyond equality – as we push forward to meet our LGBT patient's individual needs in a legal and warm locale. We help simplify same-sex couples on their family building journey by offering services that are not only accessible to them, but structured with them in mind.
>
> *(Surrogacy Mexico)*

> We are well aware of the patient 'run-around' aspects encountered by hopeful new parents when dealing with many other providers of similar services. To assure that our patients do not have to endure the non-centralized hardships encountered with most centers offering surrogacy services, our center incorporates all aspects of the gay surrogacy process into one centralized location.
>
> *(The Fertility Institutes)*

In the case of *Surrogacy Mexico*, surrogacy services are 'structured with [gay intending parents] in mind', and on *The Fertility Institutes*' website a contrast is made between other clinics that allegedly give intending parents the 'run-around' and *The Fertility Institutes* which 'incorporate all aspects of the gay surrogacy process into one centralized location'. We would suggest that to a certain degree the information outlined on this website provides an answer to the implied 'structuring' that gay intending parents are presumed to desire, namely ease of access to surrogacy services. This presumption that what gay intending parents want are surrogacy services that are simple and straightforward is also emphasized on other websites:

> In addition, surrogacy is fast, has an extremely high success rate and gives intended parents a high degree of choice and control.
>
> *(Northwest Surrogacy Center)*

> As gay intended parents, third party reproduction offers a more convenient parenting option to building tomorrow's families today. Often gay intended parents may have considered adoption as a possible option, but realize the difficulty being gay can pose on their ability to adopt.
>
> *(Surrogacy Alternatives)*

The *Northwest Surrogacy Center* website perhaps demonstrates the construction of potential clients as neoliberal repropreneurs at its most obvious, in the offer of a 'high degree of choice and control', along with the promise of an 'extremely high success rate'. These statements are paired, we would suggest, given that the good neoliberal citizen would clearly choose a clinic that is successful in delivering the promised service (i.e. a child – a good neoliberal citizen would not exercise choice and control by selecting a poorly performing service and potentially not receive the promised service). Similarly, *Surrogacy Alternatives* interpellates the neoliberal reproprenenur who wants 'convenience' (the paired contrast being with adoption, which is positioned as being either less convenient or indeed inconvenient). The following and final extract in this first mode of address demonstrates the neoliberal framing of gay men's parental desires in arguably its most blatant form on any of the websites:

> It's summer time. While the biggest worry for some of us is where to spend the next vacation, or to limit those ice cream dosages so that the bathing suit will stay intact, I would like to share with you the concern of my very proud, gay-dads-to-be friends, who have began the journey of gay surrogacy.
>
> *(Viva Family)*

In this blog entry on the *Viva Family* website, the plans of a gay couple to have a child through commercial surrogacy are listed along with forms of consumption such as choosing a vacation spot. While the author of the blog entry may not have intended to pair a child with decisions about holidays (though he or she may well have, given Krol⌀kke's (2015) work on a similar pairing with regard to egg donors), the presentation of these decisions together relies upon a neoliberal logic of consumption in which 'choices' about vacations, children and indeed how much ice cream to eat, are all indeed 'choices' to be weighed up and decided upon by the neoliberal consumer.

Across the extracts in this section, then, gay men's reproductive desires are framed by a neoliberal logic in which there is an injunction upon gay men to desire services that are 'centralized', 'structured', 'fast', 'controlled', 'convenient' and, perhaps most importantly, from which they can 'choose'. The literature on surrogacy (e.g. Krol⌀kke and Pant, 2012; Markens, 2012; Riggs, 2015b; Rudrappa, 2010), of course, has suggested that such narratives of choice are problematic when compared with the limited 'choices' often available to women who act as surrogates. Yet as we will discuss later in this chapter, rather than directly engaging with the problematic implications of the commodification of women's bodies, the websites largely appear to sidestep this by focusing on an instrumentalizing account of women who act as surrogates.

Desirability of genetic relatedness

The second mode of address that we identified highlights a concern that has been repeatedly raised in the literature on gay men and surrogacy (e.g. Dempsey, 2013; Murphy, 2015), namely the complex relationship that gay men have to normative discourses of genetic relatedness. This relationship is complex, as we suggested in Chapter 2, because while gay men are located outside the norm of reproductive heterosex, they are nonetheless interpellated into a norm in which genetic relatedness is privileged over other forms of kinship. This is not to say that a desire for genetic relatedness is the only factor driving some gay men to enter into commercial surrogacy arrangements, but it certainly appears to be a factor that shapes the decision-making of some gay men. Consequently, the emphasis on genetic relatedness on clinic websites is not surprising, as is evident in the following examples:

> Many of our LGBT clients choose surrogacy over adoption because it allows them to have a genetic relationship with the baby.
>
> *(Northwest Surrogacy Center)*

> With the assistance of an egg donor and a gestational surrogate mother, gay intended parents are provided with the ability to have children biologically related to them, as well as be recognized as the rightful and legal parents under California surrogacy and egg donation laws … By choosing the same egg donor, sharing fertilization and transferring an embryo biologically related to each male into your surrogate mother, your dream could come true together.
>
> *(Surrogacy Alternatives)*

The *Northwest Surrogacy Center* treats a desire for genetic relatedness as a taken-for-granted fact. Here a paired contrast is made between adoption and surrogacy, with the latter treated as preferable because of the potential for a genetic relationship, a distinction found in other research that reports on the accounts given by parents who have had children through commercial surrogacy (e.g. Riggs, 2015b). The *Surrogacy Alternatives* website takes this emphasis upon genetic relatedness a step further by not only emphasizing the fact that surrogacy allows for genetic relatedness, but also by proposing the idea that both men could fertilize eggs from the same donor and so both experience a genetic relationship to a child. While this practice is likely to be known among gay parenting communities (see Lewin, 2009), we would suggest it is notable that the *Surrogacy Alternatives* website specifically promotes it as a desirable option for gay intending parents, thus tapping into the idea that genetic relatedness *should* be desirable.

The following extract, although it does not specifically address the topic of genetic relatedness, implicitly supports the assumption that an *approximation* of genetic relatedness is considered desirable:

> Many gay intended parents choose an egg donor who has physical characteristics similar to the partner who is not contributing genetic material. Some look for an egg donor who shares their ethnic background.
>
> *(Circle Surrogacy)*

This extract suggests that an intending parent who will not be genetically related to the child might desire a physical resemblance that stands in for a genetic relationship. This mirrors the findings of Mamo (2005), who indicates that lesbian couples may similarly select a sperm donor who resembles the woman who will not be genetically related to the child. As Mamo suggests, such an approach to making decisions about genetic material is complex, as it both complicates how we understand relatedness in terms of physical appearance, and reinforces the desirability of visual similarities as a presumed representation of genetic similarity. This idea of 'matching' intending parents who will not be genetically related with the characteristics of donors of genetic materials also potentially serves to render invisible the role of donors themselves (i.e. by making it appear as though the child is the product solely of the two parents, as we outlined in Chapter 1). This point about rendering invisible the role of egg donors is highlighted in the final extract included in this theme:

> The surrogate or egg donor will not be present on the birth certificate unlike the few other global destinations that allow surrogacy for singles and gay couples which makes Tabasco the most appealing destination anywhere for gay surrogacy.
>
> *(Surrogacy Cancun)*

Again, while this extract does not specifically speak to genetic relatedness, we believe it is important to include as it highlights how the potential drive to approximate the norm of two genetically related parents plays out in the context of gay men and commercial surrogacy. In this extract the *Surrogacy Cancún* website uses the fact that neither women who act as surrogates nor egg donors will appear on the birth certificate, a fact that is treated as a selling point. That this should make Tabasco 'the most appealing destination' says much about what is seen as desirable by the clinic (and, potentially, gay intending parents), namely that the reproductive labour of women who act as surrogates and egg donors will not be recorded in the child's legal documents. This is a concern that we will return to later in this chapter.

Universality of the desire for a child as a marker of family

In the third and final mode of address that we identified we focus on two ideas that were frequently paired on the websites: that the desire to have a child is universal; and that families only come into existence when adults have a child. Certainly the idea that having a child is a normative feature of the life course of gay relationships is evident in the literature on gay parenting (e.g. Lewin, 2009). What is relatively unique with regard to how this plays out in the context of the clinic websites, however, is that these websites introduce the idea that a family is only made through adults having children.

In terms of the websites, the first set of extracts below demonstrates the ways in which the desire to have a child is naturalized:

> We strongly feel that the desire to have a child is a universal emotion and should not be treated with bias on the basis of ethnicity, geographical boundaries or sexual orientation.
>
> *(Baby Joy)*

> Mid-thirties, Dave is a lawyer and Jonathan is a high school teacher. They met, fell in love, decided they wanted to live happily ever after, did the thing all couples do – got married, and lived their life just like everyone else. Some days super happy, other days grumpy. It's called life. At some point they decided it was time to turn from a couple to a couple with a baby. A family.
>
> *(Viva Family)*

> Northwest Surrogacy Center, LLC helps gay intended parents create the families they have dreamed of – and the grandchildren their parents have dreamed of!
>
> *(Northwest Surrogacy Center)*

In these extracts the desire to have a child is depicted as 'a universal emotion', a 'dream', and as part of a normative relationship life course. Although these types of claims are perhaps understandable given that the websites are intended to attract potentially intended parents, the websites also function as a form of homonormativity

(Duggan, 2002) by suggesting that gay men, 'just like everyone else', should experience the desire to have a child as a 'universal emotion'. This implies that gay men who do not desire to have a child are somehow either incomplete or not 'just like everyone else'. This form of exclusion is further exemplified in the following extracts:

> A family starts with a baby. It's everyone's dream to have a baby of their own genetic relationship. Surrogacy Center Nepal (SCN) is committed to making dreams come true. SCN will treat the couples who are living together and waiting to fulfill their dream of having babies of their own.
>
> *(Surrogacy Center Nepal)*

> Having children should be a right, and not a privilege, for everybody wanting to start a family ... For many in the gay men community, surrogacy is their best option if they are looking for a fulfilling family experience.
>
> *(Surrogacy Mexico)*

The first extract reinforces claims about desire made both within this theme and the previous one (i.e. that having a child is 'everyone's dream', and specifically a child that is genetically related), in addition to making the claim that 'a family starts with a baby'. This presumption is similarly made in the second extract, which positions having children as a 'fulfilling family experience'. Again, while it is not at all surprising that these websites would normalize the desire for children (given that is what they are selling), in the process they exclude or marginalize families of choice that *do not* involve children (Weston, 1990).

In constructing children as central to family, the claims examined in this theme potentially set some gay men up for failure. In other words, if 'family starts with a baby' and having a baby is 'everyone's dream', then what happens to those gay men who, for various reasons, may be unable to have a child through surrogacy despite that being their desire (i.e. due to a pregnancy loss, infertility or economic reasons)? Furthermore, what does it mean that gay men's 'dream to have a baby of their own genetic relationship' is dependent upon the reproductive labour of others? It is to these others that we now turn to consider.

Where are the women?

In the previous sections we have referred to 'modes of address' with regard to the ways in which potential gay intending parents are hailed by surrogacy clinic websites. Through these modes of address gay men are faced with the injunction to reproduce, which is normalized through the idea that having children constitutes entry into adulthood proper, and involves the normative assumption that parents should want to be genetically related to their children. The injunction to take up these norms is enshrined in a neoliberal logic of consumption, in which gay men are positioned as agentic repropreneurs capable of taking up the call to reproduce.

Whilst, as we noted in the introduction to this chapter, it is understandable that the bulk of the website information would be directed at, and be about, intending parents, it was somewhat surprising to us that so little information was given about women who act as surrogates. Certainly in the account provided by Rudrappa and Collins (2015) it would appear that Indian clinics heavily draw upon an idealized and romanticized depiction of women who act as surrogates, depictions that function to authorize their inculcation into the capitalist logic of the clinic as money-making enterprise (i.e. by positioning them as somehow outside of commerce, or as needy recipients of the welfare of intending parents). On the websites that we examined, by contrast, the information presented to gay men rarely included mention of women who act as surrogates.

When women who act as surrogates were depicted they were primarily represented through the pairing of instrumentalization and agency. With regard to the former, women who act as surrogates were reduced to goods (thus reminiscent of our earlier point about the etymology of the word 'material'). With regard to agency, women were often simultaneously represented as service providers. This pairing is most evident in information provided on the *Growing Generations* website:

> Our Surrogates
>
> We take 1% of the women who apply to our program to become surrogates. Here is what you can expect from a GG surrogate:
>
> - Prior to meeting your surrogates she will have been fully screened medically, criminally and psychologically
> - Your surrogate will have medical insurance coverage
> - Many of our surrogates have insurance of their own that can be used for the surrogacy process
> - Surrogates in our program receive ongoing psychological support and monitoring throughout the process
> - Be matched with a surrogate that WANTS to help a gay couple or single
> - Our surrogates are financially stable and have emotional support from family and friends.

This summary provided on the website is complex, and requires close attention. The summary opens with the paternalistic claim to 'our surrogates'. Not only does the website make a possessive claim to women who act as surrogates for the clinic, but it reduces women to the singular and simplistic category of 'surrogate'. The possessive claim is further emphasized in the statement that follows, which makes reference to 'GG [*Growing Generations*] surrogate[s]', thus clearly labelling the women as properties of the clinic. Through the use of quantification rhetoric (i.e. '1%'), the clinic is able to position itself not only as possessing surrogates, but that it is discerning in its possession.

Turning to the list of characteristics, the discerning nature of the clinic is emphasized through the emphasis on screening. Yet having established women who act as surrogates as instruments in the production of a baby, the list then shifts to a focus on agency. So, as service providers, and mirroring our findings presented in Chapter 4, women who act as surrogates are expected to provide their own insurance, and to be financially stable. These, we would suggest, are contradictory claims. On the one hand, women who act as surrogates are service providers who bring with them insurance coverage. On the other hand, they are not depicted as needing an income through undertaking a surrogacy, instead being depicted as financially stable in their own right. This type of dual positioning potentially functions to implicitly mitigate concerns about the commodification of women's bodies by depicting women as not needing to do surrogacy (i.e. they are already financially stable), and thus potentially as entering into a surrogacy for altruistic, rather than financial, reasons. This echoes our arguments in Chapters 2 and 4 about what are seen as appropriately gendered orientations to love and money.

In addition to the *Growing Generations* website, two other websites made explicit mention of women who act as surrogates, with the extracts from both websites included below:

> All our surrogates stay in our own surrogate homes under our direct care & supervision.
>
> *(Baby Joy)*

> At any point in time, CSP has between 50 and 80 surrogate moms in screening, which allows us to choose the right surrogate for you.
>
> *(Center for Surrogate Parenting)*

Both of these extracts echo points made in the *Growing Generations* extract included above. In the first, women who act as surrogates are akin to properties of the clinic, under its 'direct care and supervision'. Echoing Rudrappa's (2015) findings in the Indian context, this type of regulation is treated as unproblematic and indeed as a positive for intending parents who, it would appear, are meant to be heartened by the fact that the woman carrying their child will be regulated. The second extract similarly instrumentalizes women who may potentially act as surrogates as properties of the clinic, with the depiction of 'between 50 and 80 surrogate moms in screening' evoking a Fordist imaginary of production lines and consumers selecting their preferred product. Again, the fact that this type of information is included suggests to us that clinics such as these perceive this type of information as appealing to potential intending parents, and certainly the work of Rudrappa says that this is the case.

In sum, by and large women who act as surrogates are rendered invisible in information directed at gay men on the twelve clinic websites. For those websites that did include mention of women who act as surrogates, this information was either instrumentalizing, or alluded to the agency of the women. Yet both of these, we have suggested, achieve the same end: they naturalize the labor that women undertake when carrying a child for someone else, and they sidestep the broader cultural contexts in which such naturalization occurs.

Concluding thoughts

In this chapter we have suggested that surrogacy clinic websites that target gay men arguably go beyond 'passive' advertising. Instead, they actively work to construct particular intelligible identities for gay men as reproprenenurs who are able to take up the injunction to have children to whom they are genetically related. This construction of gay men, however, is reliant upon the co-occurring marginalization and instrumentalization of women who act as surrogates. Even when claims to agency on the part of such women are evoked, these too only appear to function in the service of intending parents (i.e. to mitigate any concerns about commodification).

Whilst it is understandable, as we suggested in the introduction to this chapter, that surrogacy clinics – as businesses – would utilize advertising that is most likely to increase their revenue, our concern has been with the potential implications of this. By instrumentalizing the role of women who act as surrogates, then, intending parents are not encouraged to consider how their decisions may have consequences for the women who carry children for them. The depiction of women who act as surrogates as property of the clinic abrogates responsibility from intending parents, placing sole responsibility on clinics to manage any liabilities. As we suggested in Chapter 4, then, this type of logic does nothing to encourage a turn towards the face of the Other. If anything, the websites erase the face of the Other, suggesting instead that all that matters is the needs or desires of the neoliberal consumer.

As we have also suggested in this chapter, the sole depiction of intending parents as agentic reproprenenurs ignores the fact that success (i.e. having a baby) is not guaranteed. By implicitly discouraging any turn towards the face of the Other, we would argue, the websites are actually complicit in encouraging intending parents not to also turn towards themselves: to examine their own motivations, desires, and how they may feel if these are not fulfilled. Specifically, and as we have previously argued drawing on interview data with Australian gay men who undertook a commercial surrogacy in India (Riggs, Due & Power, 2015), the neoliberal language of 'choice' is problematic in that it may fail to prepare gay men adequately for the potential *lack* of choice they may experience. Our point here, of course, is not that gay men do not make agentic choices, nor that they are not consumers within a neoliberal marketplace. Rather, our point is that positioning them as agentic consumers fails to acknowledge that in some contexts certain decisions (such as being present at the birth or being supported in the face of a pregnancy loss) may be denied to gay men in the context of commercial surrogacy arrangements (as may also be true for heterosexual intending parents). We suggest, therefore, that whilst the framing of gay men's desire to become parents through the lens of neoliberalism is an accurate representation of the operations of reproprenenurship, it nonetheless overwrites or renders invisible the ways in which this can fail some gay men.

As such, and whilst as has been our focus throughout this book, vulnerabilities are differentially distributed across the varying parties involved in surrogacy arrangements, it seems somewhat remiss that the clinic websites are less than transparent about the particular vulnerabilities that intending parents may face. Again, this is perhaps understandable given that the primary aim of the websites is likely to attract potential customers, but it would also appear important that websites prepare potential intending parents for the full scope of what may lie ahead for them. As Martin (2015) notes, the relative lack of regulation over surrogacy services in the Americas potentially leads to a lack of oversight with regard to the particular concerns that we raise here. The question of oversight is one that we will take up in the following chapter in which we focus on media and legislative responses to surrogacy.

Moving beyond the specific findings of this chapter and returning to the broader analytic frameworks of this book as introduced in Chapter 1, a final note is necessary with regard to the face of the Other. Throughout much of this book we have focused on individual parties involved in surrogacy arrangements. Beyond these individual parties, however, there is the issue of the planet itself, and the sustainability of human life at current growth rates. Certainly the blame for environmental abuses or the unsustainability of population growth cannot be laid at the door of those who enter into surrogacy arrangements, nor those who facilitate them (i.e. clinics). Yet this does not mean that caution is not warranted with regard to the pursuit of human life at any cost, including the cost to human children already alive who cannot live with their birth parents, and for whom statutory child protection agencies are often inadequate. The face of the Other in the form of the planet and all that lives on it, then, constitutes part of the larger picture in which surrogacy clinics operate. That such clinics contribute to population growth and do so within a capitalist logic is not something that can be ignored, even if we might wish to stop short of laying the blame on clinics. Rather, our point in closing this chapter with these remarks is to encourage further reflection on how surrogacy clinics are complicit with pronatalism, and how in turn pronatalism is part of a larger concern about what is done in the name of humanity, and at the cost of whom (including the planet and other species).

A critical health approach to the issues we have raised in these concluding thoughts, then, must go beyond examining individual health disparities and individual engagements with the operations of capitalism. The health of societies and indeed the planet and all that lives on it are intimately enmeshed with the wellbeing of individuals. Certainly, halting surrogacy arrangements is not going to provide a significant response to population growth given the relatively small contribution that such arrangements make. At the same time, however, the whole-hearted acceptance of surrogacy in certain quarters (even if not in others) is part of a broader cultural naturalization of reproduction at any cost, just as is the naturalization of the ways in which particular people's lives and bodies are seen as open to instrumentalization (which mirrors, as we suggested in Chapter 2, the instrumentalization of the lives and bodies of other species). Engaging in a critique of the logic informing surrogacy, as we do in this book, is part of a broader mode of critique focused on the cultural production of inequalities that are premised upon the over-valuing of particular worldviews.

7

MEDIA AND PUBLIC DISCOURSE

Overview

In this chapter we consider two sources of representation with regard to surrogacy: that seen in the mainstream media, and that seen in submissions to an Australian inquiry concerning surrogacy law reform. We focus in this chapter on representations of transnational surrogacy since it is this form of surrogacy arrangement that typically attracts the most attention in mainstream consciousness: an interesting point in itself. As argued throughout this book thus far, the practice of surrogacy (either commercial or altruistic) brings with it a range of often competing discourses, and these will shape public understanding of surrogacy (Van den Akker, Camara & Hunt, 2016; Shalev & Lemish, 2011; Millbank, 2012). As such, the analysis of public representations of surrogacy is useful for what it tells us about the position of surrogacy more broadly in public consciousness. Furthermore, public representations of surrogacy can be seen as a starting point for considering ways forward, as discussed in the next chapter.

In terms of media coverage concerning transnational surrogacy, research suggests that such coverage is increasing (Van den Akker et al., 2016; Shalev & Lemish, 2011). Researchers have suggested that this increase in media coverage may relate to the ways in which surrogacy represents a departure from family arrangements which are considered normative, with surrogacy challenging understandings of kinship, as argued in the first two chapters of this book (see Van den Akker et al., 2016; Shalev & Lemish, 2011). As such, surrogacy may be seen to represent a particularly 'newsworthy' topic (Markens, 2007), particularly when it involves extreme stories such as those relating to child abuse or arrangements for care of a child which are not clear or which break down – such as the Baby M case (Van den Akker et al., 2016; Markens, 2007). Nevertheless, as Susan Markens argues, the volume of media coverage of surrogacy appears to exceed that which could be expected on the basis of the incidence of surrogacy arrangements themselves.

Given the volume of media reports on surrogacy, there is a growing field of research exploring media depictions of both transnational surrogacy (e.g. Fixmer-Oraiz, 2013; Crawshaw, Purewal & Van den Akker, 2013; Riggs & Due, 2013; Markens, 2007, 2012) and altruistic surrogacy (e.g. Van den Akker et al., 2016). This previous research has indicated that surrogacy – whether commercial or altruistic – is generally reported within a negative framework in the media, and that this has been the case since the 1980s when coverage of surrogacy first began to occur in the media (Dunn, Ryan & O'Brien, 1988; Halman, Abbey & Andrews, 1992; Krishnan, 1994; Poote & Van den Akker, 2009; Suzuki, Hoshi, Minai, Yanaihara, Takeda & Yamagata, 2006; Markens, 2012), although the 'tone' of the coverage has been found to vary depending on the sexual orientation of the intending parents and the precise circumstances in which an arrangement is made (Murphy, 2015; Millbank, 2012). Regardless, analysis of the increasing media coverage of surrogacy is important since, as Michelle Imison and Steven Schweinsberg (2013) argue, the mainstream media is central to the general public's understanding of transnational surrogacy. Moreover, knowledge concerning dominant representations of surrogacy may help to shed light on attitudinal responses to surrogacy itself (Crawshaw et al., 2013), and has the potential to either directly or indirectly inform law reform (Millbank, 2012).

While there is a body of research that has explored media representations of surrogacy, less research has considered representations of surrogacy in political discourse. In her analysis of Australia media and parliamentary representations of surrogacy, Jenni Millbank (2012) found similar discourses in both sources of representation, as explored further below, suggesting that the two are closely related. Moreover, she found that in both contexts, discourses of 'naturalness', family and genetics were used to justify positions both advocating for *and* against potential law reforms concerning surrogacy in Australian. Importantly, she suggests that her analysis of these two sources indicates that members of parliament are informed by media coverage of surrogacy at least to some degree, further highlighting the importance of considering media discourse when considering surrogacy and its implications for the health and wellbeing of all parties.

Below, we outline the specific findings of the previous research mentioned above, before turning to an analysis of media and political discourse concerning surrogacy in Australia. Specifically, we explore media representations of intending parents engaging in transnational surrogacy arrangements, media representations of the case of Baby Gammy in the Australian mainstream media, as well as public submissions to the inquiry that preceded the passing of the New South Wales *Surrogacy Bill (2010)*.

Public discourses about surrogacy

Previous research concerning representations of surrogacy in the media has found a diverse range of discourses and tropes. However, one common thread through most of the literature in this area is the finding that most coverage of surrogacy is alarmist. This is the case even in relation to altruistic surrogacy, with research by Olga Van den Akker and colleagues (2016) concerning altruistic surrogacy in the United Kingdom finding that newspapers were more likely to report on surrogacy when there was an emotional element to report – particularly in relation to alarmist coverage. Specifically, newspapers typically reported altruistic surrogacy through a framework of loss, and framed intending parents' 'need' for surrogacy in terms of vulnerability (see also Riggs & Due, 2013). Moreover, most of the coverage examined by Van den Akker and colleagues focused on social and legal issues, with very few media outlets discussing medical details for either the intending parents or the woman acting as a surrogate, with the latter being all but invisible in the media reports they examined.

Similarly, the relative invisibility of women who act as surrogates was found in Australian research on media coverage of transnational surrogacy conducted by Imison and Schweinsberg (2013). Imison and Schweinsberg examined Australian mainstream news media coverage of medical tourism – including people travelling for international surrogacy arrangements – to low- and middle-income countries. They found that 'access to services' was the most evident theme in the media they analysed, with sub-themes of the low costs of services overseas, being able to 'feel good', the opportunity to travel and lower waiting times than in Australia. 'Credibility' was a common trope, with personal stories, images and specific details such as numbers of clients or details of services all being used to lend credence to reporting on medical tourism and to personalize stories according to individual circumstances. The final theme found was that of risk. In particular, 'ethical dilemmas' were commonly seen, as was discussion of the safety of particular procedures, countries or practitioners. On the whole, Imison and Schweinsberg (2013) note that Australian media coverage tends to focus specifically on the experiences of Australian individuals undertaking medical tourism, rather than broader issues with medical tourism in low- and middle-income countries. They note, in particular, that there was very little media attention given to 'those who make … medical tourism possible, such as surrogate mothers and organ donors' (p. 10). Moreover, they note that such representations are consumer-focused, and push other issues involved in medical tourism aside as less newsworthy (i.e. the ethics of medical tourism).

Discourses of consumerism have also been found in Australian research by Murphy (2015) and research in the United States by Markens (2012). For example, Murphy analysed media coverage of gay male intending parents in both Australia and the United States. His analyses focused on media representations of the men themselves, finding that in both contexts they were typically represented as 'choosing' surrogacy rather than being 'forced' to use surrogacy arrangements due to medical infertility (as was the case for representations of heterosexual couples). Murphy argues that such discourses of choice are pronounced since the media he examined represented gay male couples as outside the normative family structure, and unlikely to experience the 'drive' to have children that heterosexual couples are presumed to have (similar to a point we made in Chapter 5 with regard to children's storybooks). As such, Murphy found that discourses of choice and consumption were most evident in the media coverage he analysed, whereby consumerist narratives (e.g. 'shopping') were privileged over narratives of desire or personalization. Specifically, media coverage in both Australia and the United States focused on the cost involved in transnational surrogacy arrangements, citing specific details such as clinic costs as rhetorical devices to support consumerist discourses. Nevertheless, Murphy notes that despite these discourses, male intending parents were still represented more frequently than the women who act as surrogates for them, who were typically overlooked.

Whilst in the Australian context Murphy (2015) implicitly suggests that media portrayals of gay men are negative in their focus on consumerism, Joanna Gondouin (2012) discusses a positive portrayal of a gay couple in her analysis of a Swedish documentary series, *Children at all Costs*, which examined the couple and their surrogacy arrangements in India. Gondouin found that the couple were personalized through their portrayal in the documentary, particularly through representations of family and discourses of vulnerability, innocence and generosity – with the latter depicted specifically as generosity towards the woman acting as a surrogate in India. Interestingly, and unlike in most other research (e.g. Van den Akker et al., 2016), Gondouin notes that *Children at all Costs* does spend time on representations of the woman acting as a surrogate, although these representations are not as favourable as those of the intending parents.

While much of the literature concerning surrogacy has focused on commodification, as noted in the first two chapters of this book, discourses of commodification have not been commonly reported in research on media representations concerning surrogacy. One exception to this is research by Markens (2007, 2012). For example, in a paper examining US media coverage of surrogacy, Markens (2012) discusses several blogs and editorials written from within the United States, which provide detailed coverage of surrogacy in terms of the potential to commodify women's bodies, drawing on rhetoric representing surrogacy as perpetuating inequalities, as exploitative and as responsible for the commercialization of children. Markens discusses the dilemmatic nature of these discourses of global labour, noting that other media outlets draw on and reproduce discourses of opportunity through positive framings of the outcomes of transnational surrogacy arrangements for women in low- and middle-income countries.

Research by Charlotte Kroløkke and colleagues (2010) suggests that public discourse surrounding surrogacy is often framed in two distinct ways concerning choice, reflecting the binary of altruistic and commercial surrogacy. Within the former, women who act as surrogates are portrayed as having the capacity to bestow a 'gift'. Kroløkke and colleagues suggest that such portrayals are highly gender normative, with women who act as surrogates referred to in terms such as 'goddess', 'giver' and with pregnancy itself depicted as a 'calling', reflecting our discussion of gendered labour in Chapter 2. By contrast, women who act as commercial surrogates are often depicted as mercenary *non*-maternal women who happily relinquish 'their' babies for others; with this dichotomy between love and money seen also in discussions of women who choose to act as surrogates in Chapter 3. From this perspective, women who act as surrogates are depicted as workers doing a job, one that is free from emotional labour and which, as a result, translates into the depiction of women who act as commercial surrogates as heartless and easily able to relinquish the child that they carry (see also Teman, 2010).

In our research on media representation of surrogacy (Riggs & Due, 2010), we found that while media outlets may not specifically draw on discourses of commodification in their representations of surrogacy, discourses which position women acting as surrogates in low- and middle-income countries as standing to gain financially from surrogacy arrangements can be read as potentially endorsing commodification. We have further suggested (Riggs & Due, 2013) that metaphors of surrogacy as a 'business' or 'industry' are common in the Australian media coverage of surrogacy, leading to significant differences in the representations of women who act as surrogates and intending parents. In particular, we noted that intending parents are portrayed as free to undertake reproductive travel, while women in India are positioned as fixed producers of goods within a reproductive economy.

In terms of political representations, both Millbank (2012) and Markens (2007) demonstrate how parliamentary responses and debate concerning surrogacy can potentially stem from media coverage. For example, Markens (2007) examined parliamentary and media responses to the Baby M case, indicating that media coverage of this particular breakdown of custody following the birth of a baby through a surrogacy arrangement was a driving factor in bringing surrogacy to the attention of legislators in New York State. In addition, Markens (2007) notes that the framing of media coverage was directly related to specific policy responses. She highlights how framing which discussed social justice and the right to parenthood typically advocated for legal and regulated surrogacy practices. As an example, she notes how framing which pitched surrogacy as 'baby selling' advocated for bans.

In the Australian context, Millbank (2012) has found that arguments made by politicians concerning surrogacy and potential law reform directly mirror those seen in the media, reflecting the work of Markens (2007) discussed above. Millbank suggests that politicians draw from both personal experiences and the media to inform their debate, rather than evidence such as that derived from empirical studies concerning the outcomes of surrogacy arrangements. In terms of the specific discourse she found, Millbank notes that one of the main potential drivers of law reform to make surrogacy more accessible in Australia appeared in discourses of family formation and fertility. In particular, she found discourses of 'naturalistic' maternal desire in both parliamentary debates and media representations, with this desire being privileged over consideration for the precise method of reproduction. Reflecting the work of Murphy (2015) in relation to his media analysis, Millbank also found that naturalizing discourses were typically seen only in relation to heterosexual couples (and specifically women) and were not extended to gay couples.

The point at which discourses diverge in media representations compared to parliamentary debates is with regard to the question of payment. Specifically,

Millbank found that parliamentarians were opposed to commercial surrogacy, whereas media representations do not either privilege or dismiss payment – instead subsuming discussion of payment to a woman acting as a surrogate within the discourse of relationality, for example such that she came to be seen as part of an extended family.

Media and public inquiry analysis

In our analysis below we explore:

1 media coverage of intending parents involved in transnational commercial surrogacy arrangements (specifically surrogacy in India);
2 Australian media coverage of the Baby Gammy case; and
3 public submissions related to the New South Wales *Surrogacy Bill* which passed in 2010.

Data for representations of both Baby Gammy and transnational commercial surrogacy arrangements were sourced from Australian newspapers and online news sources with the highest readership and circulation, as identified by the Australian Press Council's *State of News Print Media 2007* report. These papers and their online news counterparts are: the *Herald Sun*, the *Daily Telegraph*, *The Courier-Mail*, *Sydney Morning Herald*, *The Age*, *The West Australian*, *The Australian*, *The Advertiser*, *The Financial Review*, *The Mercury*, *The Canberra Times* and the *N.T. News*. In relation to Baby Gammy, the search term 'Baby gammy OR gammy' were put into Factiva for the time period of July to December 2014 when media coverage was at its peak. For transnational surrogacy, the search term 'surrog* AND India' was used, and media articles were sourced from newspapers published between 1 January 2009 and December 2016, due to the fact that a Google Insights search indicated that the search term 'surrogacy India' went from no searches prior to 2009, to over 100 searches made from within Australia in early 2009. The search for Baby Gammy returned 127 relevant media articles, while the search for transnational surrogacy returned 296 relevant articles.

Finally, we analyse public representations of surrogacy as seen through submission to the public inquiry that preceded the passing of the *Surrogacy Bill (2010)* by the parliament of the Australian state of New South Wales on 10 November 2010. Notably, whilst the primary focus of the inquiry that informed the Bill (Robertson, 2009) was on altruistic surrogacy, issues related to commercial surrogacy were repeatedly referred to within submissions to the inquiry, and commercial surrogacy became a large part of the Bill, with the introduction of an amendment to the Bill that prohibited transnational commercial surrogacy undertaken by any resident of the state.

Intending parents, reproductive vulnerability and agency

In this first analytic section, we explore media representations of intending parents involved in commercial surrogacy arrangements, particularly with regard to what we have elsewhere termed their 'reproductive vulnerability' (Riggs & Due, 2013). Specifically, we explore how an inability to conceive via reproductive heterosex renders intending parents vulnerable; a vulnerability that they may seek to overcome through surrogacy. Moreover, as we shall see, this potential vulnerability of intending parents is typically mitigated in the media through reference to 'intent', which as we argued in Chapter 1 serves to assert the desires of intending parents over any other parties.

In the first example – a newspaper article by Marriner (2012) – we see how the media touch on reproductive vulnerability, only then to use the notion of 'intent' to make vulnerability disappear. Specifically, the article draws upon emotive language in order to explore intending parents' decisions to undertake commercial surrogacy, and the associated potential for reproductive vulnerability. This emotion is particularly evoked through references to the 'fertility profile' of the female partner (Ms Wylie) and the tyranny of distance associated with international surrogacy ('The hardest part of overseas surrogacy was not the $80,000 they spent, she said, but the detachment of distance'). Yet this narrative of vulnerability concerning fertility and travel is preceded in the article by describing the decision to engage in commercial surrogacy as a 'big leap of faith', and descriptions of the Wylies' child as 'living proof' of their 'bond' to India (where the couple undertook surrogacy). Thus whilst the couple's reproductive vulnerability is referred to, it is framed in terms of 'overcoming an obstacle', and this overcoming provides not simply a child, but also a bond to another country. Interestingly, this notion of a 'bond' is not framed as a product of reproductive vulnerability per se (i.e. that there is a bond because surrogacy in India addressed the couple's infertility), but rather as a response to a 'gift' relationship; specifically, Ms Wylie is quoted as saying of the woman who acted as a surrogate: 'we feel [that our child] is a gift [the surrogate] gave us'.

Emotive descriptions of intending parents are seen again in an article published in the *Herald Sun* in 2011, which discusses the 'joy' experienced by an Australian gay couple after realizing their 'dream' of having male twins through a surrogacy arrangement. After outlining the joy they experienced after initially feeling nervous with their twin boys, the article goes on to state:

> they had resigned themselves to the fact they were not going to have children. But [Tony] said they desperately wanted a family of their own …
>
> Melbourne family psychologist Sally-Anne McCormack said … 'They were clearly desperate to have children and there are people who have children who don't have that same passion'.
>
> *(Herald Sun, 2011)*

Here, the article draws upon emotive language to build up a case that legitimates transnational surrogacy arrangements by positioning such arrangements as solutions to a problem, thus positioning the couple as agentic, rather than vulnerable. This can be seen in the use of a causal narrative (i.e. resignation to not having children leading to desperation and then to surrogacy as the solution), as well as the use of expert voicing in the final section (where a psychologist explicitly positions the couple as active in their decision to enter into a surrogacy arrangement in order to have children). Again, then, the reproductive vulnerabilities of the intending parents are put aside in favour of a narrative of intent to have a child; a subject position which ultimately accords them agency.

Also of interest to us is the way in which describing surrogacy in terms of joy and dreams (versus the language of 'desperation') highlights what disappears when reproductive vulnerabilities are treated as plot narratives or as problems to be overcome. In the case of the report considered above, part of what disappears is the fact that gay men in Australia occupy an inherently vulnerable position in terms of children, because (at least for cisgender gay men) they cannot carry children themselves, combined with the fact that historically legislation in Australia has prevented gay men from having children other than through privately negotiating co-parenting relationships with women (van Reyk, 2007). In this sense, gay men's reproductive vulnerabilities represent the very nexus of how the state produces such vulnerabilities (where having children is represented as desirable, but where having children is rendered legally impossible), yet in the news report such vulnerabilities are made to disappear.

As such, to experience joy through the fulfilment of a dream is an entirely expected response for gay men who historically may have felt no avenues open to them. Yet what potentially disappears here when 'desperation' becomes a mere precursor to 'joy' is that the desires that fuel such desperation are not treated seriously. In other words, we would suggest that there is a significant difference between prohibition and desire, and that whilst the former might fuel the latter, once the former is removed (as is the case for gay men who now, in most Australian states, can undertake transnational surrogacy, can in all Australian states enter onshore altruistic surrogacy arrangements, can in all states undertake onshore adoption, and can in all states enter into long-term foster care arrangements), what remains is reproductive vulnerability. In other words, what shapes some gay men's desires to have children who are genetically related to them (and the factors that still bar that even with decreased prohibition) is thus left unmentioned. As a result, the net effects of the 'desperation' are left unexplored.

The following and final article considered in this section also highlights how vulnerabilities in regard to commissioning parents are raised, only to be swept away through a focus on their location as agentic consumers by virtue of their intent to have a child. This article, by Barlass (2011), highlights the vulnerabilities of the intending parents in terms of their desire to have a child by reference to failed previous attempts at IVF with a woman acting as a surrogate, and by outlining the couple's decision to cease surrogacy attempts due to costs. However, the article goes on to state that the couple in question – the Gearys – decided to make a 'last ditch effort', which led to a successful pregnancy. Despite recognition of their reliance upon transnational surrogacy and the vulnerability this represents, the article primarily presents the Gearys as agentic consumers, particularly through reference to their ability to make decisions about their desire to pursue surrogacy, and to travel if they wished.

Furthermore, and following their 'success', the Gearys' vulnerabilities are further hidden through the representation of the couple as holding the power in their relationship to the surrogate. For example, the article quotes Mrs Geary as saying, in reference to the woman who acted as a surrogate for the couple: 'I would take Mia [baby] down to see her or she would bring the milk she expressed in. I would invite her to sit down and give her Mia to hold.' Here, it is Mrs Geary who holds the ability to offer 'invitations' to 'their' surrogate, who clearly does not hold a similar power to offer invitations for a relationship. Yet at the same time, it is the surrogate who expresses the milk, and it is the surrogate to whom the Gearys show gratitude. As such, whilst much of the language of the article appears to introduce a shift away from any vulnerability on the part of the Gearys, their vulnerability within a global reproductive market continues to show through. Our point of course is not that the Gearys were necessarily any more vulnerable than was the woman who acted as their surrogate, but rather that vulnerabilities within the context of reproductive travel exist for all parties. Nevertheless, media representations of people involved in surrogacy arrangements typically either discount vulnerabilities altogether, or emphasize them only in the case of women acting as surrogates. Further examples of vulnerability in the representation of women acting as surrogates can be seen in the following section concerning representations of the controversy surrounding Baby Gammy.

Women who act as surrogates: visible yet vulnerable

As mentioned briefly in the previous chapter, the Baby Gammy case involved an Australian heterosexual couple (Wendy and David Farnell) who requested that a Thai woman acting as a surrogate for them abort one of the twins she was carrying after finding out that the child had Down syndrome. The woman acting as a surrogate – Pattharamon Chanbua (alternately spelt 'Janbua' in the media) – refused. When the twins (a girl and a boy – with the boy child in question later named 'Gammy') were seven months old, the Farnells travelled to Thailand and took the girl to Australia but left Gammy with Ms Chanbua. While this caused a media scandal in its own right, further controversy arose when the media released details of Mr Farnell's past imprisonment for the sexual abuse of young girls: a revelation which prompted Ms Chanbua to also request custody of the girl taken by the Farnells. The case led to widespread investigation of Thai surrogacy clinics by Thai officials, including raids and new regulations (Cohen, 2015), and eventually the closure of commercial surrogacy within Thailand to foreign citizens.

Unlike much of the previous research noted above, which found that the media rarely provided details about women acting as surrogates themselves, the Australian media coverage of Baby Gammy did provide specific details concerning Pattharamon

Chanbua. Indeed, representations of the situation of Ms Chanbua were one of the most common themes in this coverage, and often served to highlight the apparent dangers of transnational commercial surrogacy. An example of this is seen in an article by Murdoch (2014). The article portrays the events surrounding Baby Gammy in a manner consistent with the 'alarmist' coverage noted by Van den Akker and colleagues (2016) in their research on media representations of surrogacy in the United Kingdom. Similar to articles mentioned in the previous sections, the events of the Baby Gammy case are described in the Murdoch article through the use of emotive language, citing specific details particularly in relation to Ms Chanbua's understandings of the arrangement, including her concerns about how she would become pregnant. For example, the article quotes Ms Chanbua as saying 'I asked the agency, "Did I have to sleep with the man?" I was an innocent young girl'. Arguably, these details serve to position Ms Chanbua as both vulnerable and exploited.

However, it is notable that Ms Chanbua's voice was represented at all in the media coverage of this incident since, as noted in the previous section and summary of previous literature above, representations of women who act as surrogates in the media appear to be rare (Imison & Schweinsberg, 2013; Murphy, 2015). It is notable, then, that the Australian media coverage surrounding Baby Gammy frequently reported quotes from Ms Chanbua. In this article, and many others like it, Ms Chanbua is represented through first-person narratives, presumably as a result of either an interview or a press release (this is unclear from the article itself). In particular, Ms Chanbua is represented as struggling and innocent (e.g. she is quoted as saying 'my husband agreed [to the surrogacy arrangement] because we didn't have money to pay our debt and I didn't need to have sex with another man'), and therefore presumably at risk of exploitation. Indeed, the theme of potential exploitation runs throughout this article, including through references to threats made by the Farnells to Ms Chanbua, particularly in relation to potential non-payment.

This representation of Ms Chanbua as both vulnerable and potentially at risk of exploitation is particularly interesting since previous research (e.g. Kroløkke et al., 2010) has generally found that women involved in commercial surrogacy arrangements are presented as mercenary and 'unmotherly'. Here, the representation of Ms Chanbua's apparent 'innocence' and her decision to stand up to pressure to abort the twins (e.g. 'They told me to have an abortion but I didn't agree because I am afraid of sin') works to present her as a 'good mother' (Maushart, 1997), a point we take up further in the conclusion of this chapter. On the other hand, Ms Chanbua is not represented as similarly able to overcome her vulnerability – particularly since she remains vulnerable by virtue of poverty and the need for donations.

Despite representations of Ms Chanbua's vulnerability, it is nonetheless notable that the media reports of the case portray the story largely from the perspective of Ms Chanbua herself. Again, this represents an interesting departure from the findings of previous research, which has typically found that media reports focus primarily or solely on intending parents (e.g. Murphy, 2015). A further example is provided in the following extract:

> Cash-strapped surrogate mother Pattharamon Janbua, 21, and her husband were paid $16,000 by the couple … On finding out that the unborn child had Down syndrome, they initially pressed for an abortion.
>
> *(King, 2014)*

Both this article and the one previously discussed provide specific details of the surrogacy arrangement, including details concerning payment and other costs. This coverage reflects the findings of Imison and Schweinsberg (2013), who similarly note that media coverage of surrogacy frequently provides specific details or arrangements to lend credibility to stories – and we would suggest that in addition, such coverage serves to position surrogacy firmly within the logic of capitalism through the focus on the exchange of goods and services. Moreover, specific details regarding costs allow the media to claim intimate knowledge of the arrangements, thereby presenting coverage which may be subjective in a way which appears factual – a point which has particular ramifications given who is presented as vulnerable and who is not. Indeed, the costs discussed in these articles position Ms Chanbua as exploited by the Farnells by virtue of the small amounts she was paid. This is particularly seen in the above extract, where the details of the initial payment are provided directly before the revelations that Ms Chanbua was subsequently 'pressed' to have an abortion. Again, the representations of Ms Chanbua as exploited and vulnerable are particularly interesting given that in fact she apparently resisted pressure at several stages in the pregnancy: including in relation to having an abortion, and in relation to keeping Gammy. While the exact facts of the case are unknown, the fact that the media chose to represent Ms Chanbua within a framework of vulnerability rather than of agency is of note.

Interestingly, this article follows the details of the surrogacy arrangement with a quote from Sam Everingham (President of *Surrogacy Australia*). The quote provides a good example of Marken's (2007) argument that media framings are closely related to specific positions in relation to policy or legislative reform. Specifically, Mr Everingham is quoted as highlighting the shock of the story for many intending parents in Australia who have been unsuccessful with IVF or who are medically infertile, and notes that they are 'having to go overseas because the Australian system is failing them'. Everingham's comments at the end of the article therefore position intending parents and the need for surrogacy in terms of medical infertility, thereby paving the way for calls for less restrictive surrogacy laws. Indeed, the final dominant theme seen in media coverage of the Baby Gammy case was the failure of the system overall to protect the rights of all people involved in surrogacy arrangements – although this coverage was divided in terms of any suggestions for law reform. This is seen in the following extract, taken from one of the earliest reports concerning the incident:

> Recent revelations … shed a rare light on the hidden and fundamentally unjust world of international commercial surrogacy … Australia recognises the dangers of commercial surrogacy: throughout this country it is illegal to

> enter into any arrangement that compensates the surrogate for anything more than out-of-pocket expenses.
>
> *(Gallagher, 2014)*

This article positions surrogacy in such as way as to advocate for restrictions on commercial surrogacy in Australia, and for all states in Australia to use the criminal justice system to discourage intending parents to enter commercial surrogacy arrangements transnationally. This argument is built up particularly through explicit reference to commercial surrogacy as 'unjust'. After positioning surrogacy in this way, the article goes on to further justify its position by representing Ms Chanbua as exploited (e.g. stating that she was 'used so badly' and describing her as 'barely out of her teens'). Moreover, and unlike the previous extract, this extract positions the Farnells as firmly in the wrong (that is, through their alleged exploitation of Ms Chanbua), rather than as victims of surrogacy legislation which forces them overseas. Again, this is a notable representation given that the previous section found that intending parents were represented in a framework of vulnerability and agency – with vulnerability often seen as specifically in response to situations which 'force' them overseas. Indeed, the article continues to specifically suggest that while many intended parents have 'good intentions', others do not, hence the dangers of commercial surrogacy. As such, this article appears to accord intending parents agency but not vulnerability – almost a reversal of the representations seen in the previous section.

Inquiry submissions: normative constructions of women

Inquiries such as that which led to the *Surrogacy Bill (2010)* typically produce a large amount of publicly available documentation. In the case of the New South Wales Standing Committee on Law and Justice's inquiry into *Legislation on Altruistic Surrogacy in NSW*, there were forty submissions made by members of the public, including academics, parents by surrogacy and professional bodies. There were also four public hearings in which these groups could present further information. The inquiry itself produced a report (Robertson, 2009), and this was discussed on two separate occasions by members of the New South Wales Legislative Committee. The subsequent Bill was then read into parliament and debated, and then two days later an amendment was introduced and the Bill was discussed again and then passed.

Data analysed in this section are thirty-nine of the forty public submissions made to the inquiry. All bar one of the submissions are freely available on the Standing Committee's website (the remaining submission, #13, was confidential and thus not published on the website). The reason for selecting this particular data set was that it contains a diverse range of viewpoints from across a range of stakeholders. The discussions of the report and the readings of the Bill, whilst interesting in their own right, only include the representations of surrogacy endorsed by members of parliament, and thus are not necessarily representative of the broader public. The evidence given at public hearings, whilst often including a somewhat broader spread of viewpoints from the general public, still tended towards privileging academic standpoints and information provided by professionals in the field of surrogacy. We thus consider it appropriate to focus on the public submissions in order to canvas the widest range of opinions within any of the forms of data available in regard to the inquiry.

In relation to public discourse about surrogacy as represented by the inquiry, of particular interest is the fact that the construction of women and motherhood in many of the submissions simultaneously devalued women who act as surrogates, whilst also frequently arguing for their status as the child's 'proper' mother. These seemingly opposing ideological accounts of surrogacy are, we argue, dilemmatic in the sense outlined by Billig (1999), who proposes that not only are ideological positions typically contradictory, but that none of the options available within a given ideology are inherently positive or non-normalizing. With these observations in mind, our interest in this section is to explore how the bodies, roles and identities of women who act as surrogates were constructed within submissions made to the inquiry.

As is often the case in debates over reproduction and families, many of the submissions to the inquiry evoked the notion of children's 'best interests' to argue for a particular viewpoint. The particular evocation of this argument that appeared repeatedly in the submissions was one in which it was presumed that all children:

1 need a mother;
2 are damaged by not knowing a mother; and
3 that a child's 'true' mother is the woman who carries them from conception to birth.

In many instances this line of argument was justified through recourse to religious claims, such as is the case in the first extract below. However, what lies at the heart of these claims is a normative notion of motherhood, as is exemplified by the extract below:

> Because of the person's innate dignity, the truly responsible procreation of the unborn child must be the fruit of marriage. In other words, the spouses conceive a child only through their reciprocal self-giving; they become a father and a mother only through each other... It is difficult enough for a child to come to terms with being abandoned by his/her parents. Many of these children suffer for years, often blaming themselves, and trying to make contact with the parent/parents who, he believes, abandon him ... How much worse would it be for a child to learn that the mother who gave him birth, either a genetic stranger, who did not love him but merely hosted him in her womb, or a mother genetically related to him, bore him, not out of love for him but simply to give him away to someone else. It is a tragedy not to be loved by one's parents, particularly by one's mother. For the State to legally sanction this is monstrous and cruel.
>
> *(Family Life International, Ms Gail Instance, Submission #16)*

This extract introduces three key threads that run through many of the submissions made to the inquiry. The first thread is one in which surrogacy is depicted as the 'worst' form of family making (i.e. 'monstrous and cruel') by comparison to other forms that are also treated as bad (i.e. children who are 'abandoned') and of course by comparison with the ideal form of family making (i.e. 'the fruit of marriage').

As seen in Chapter 3, the second thread is one in which women who act as surrogates are by default referred to as mothers, yet at the same time they are treated as always already being *failed* mothers. In the first extract above, to love a child is not to carry them and give them away, but rather it is to carry them and raise them. Women who carry children, but who 'give [them] away to someone else', are depicted still as 'mothers', but they are depicted as inadequate *women* (i.e. 'merely hosted', 'simply to give away', 'not out of love'). Here the emotional labour that goes into, and the motivations that underpin, surrogacy are rendered invisible through the idealization of what a 'mother' should be and want.

Finally, this extract epitomizes the adult-centric nature of the arguments presented in many of the submissions in terms of the 'best interests of the child'. Not only are the claims made in this extract obviously premised upon a heteronormative view of families, but they are also premised upon one in which it is mothers and fathers who accord an identity to one another, rather than the categories of mother and father only making sense in relation to children. In other words, whilst in the extract much is made of the 'tragedy not to be loved by one's parents', such an account is entirely adult-centric in its orientation: it displays no capacity to consider what children actually need or want, and instead capitulates to a highly normative understanding of children in which they are always and ever the product of the desires of others, rather than also being subjects who through their very being make the categories 'mother' and 'father' intelligible.

In the following extract the reification of a very particular image of 'the maternal' is rendered even more clearly:

> Any legislative changes must consider the physiological, emotional, and psychological processes that occurring during any pregnancy, irrespective of the origins of the sperm and/or ova. Proponents of surrogacy, altruistic or otherwise have claimed that the surrogate mother is merely an incubator in the process, which implies that a pregnant woman is an inanimate object void of any physiological, emotional or psychological responses to being pregnant. This view diminishes the role of women and demeans the human responses to motherhood and the birthing process. Legislators must therefore give due consideration to the normal attachment and bonding processes that occur between a mother and her unborn child and the child to its mother, and closely examine the potential and/or lasting effects that may result for both, if or when these factors are ignored.
>
> *(Vanish, Ms Patricia Lauria, Submission #6)*

In this extract a sympathetic view of women who act as surrogates is endorsed. Yet in order to warrant this claim, the extract relies upon a highly normative notion of motherhood, one in which 'normal attachment and bonding processes that occur between a mother and her unborn child' are treated as universal and unquestionable. This leads us to suggest that whilst the tenor of the extract is one in which women's bodies are the key issue of concern (and to a lesser degree the impact of surrogacy on children), the actual standpoint endorsed within the extract only serves to reify motherhood as always being the same for all women, a powerful discourse that has long been challenged (e.g. see chapters in Nathanson & Tuley, 2009).

Importantly for our argument in this book, the type of claim about mothers made in the extract above does nothing to actually examine the structural inequities that require attention in regards to the ethics of surrogacy, and instead diverts our attention to an idealized image of motherhood that is not simply potentially unproductive for some women who act as surrogates and the children they bear, but perhaps more importantly for all women who feel compelled to 'normally attach and bond' to their children. In sum, a major theme seen in submissions to the inquiry – and seen in the extracts above – included not only opposition to surrogacy itself, but more also a commitment to a highly normative understanding of mothering.

Turning now to examine submissions that were supportive of surrogacy, it is important to acknowledge that there was less consistency amongst these submissions (and there were less of these overall in comparison to those which spoke against surrogacy). What did appear to repeat in the submissions in support of surrogacy, however, reiterated the previous literature on representations of surrogacy, namely the depiction of it as a gift, as can be seen in the following extract:

> Please, don't deliberate on this issue – there are so many loving and caring people in this state alone who wish to make another person a part of that loving environment – how can we let bureaucracy and red tape stop that? Why is there a difference for a willing person to offer you the most wonderful gift in the world, to a young teenage mother to bring life to something that may not be wanted? It's simply not fair! Life deals us cards that can sometimes be a little hard to deal with and this is one of them. With the right law in place and the right guidelines to ensure that the child's wellbeing is always at the forefront of any decision, why can't this be a simple process? This is not merely moneymaking scheme by welcome uteruses – it's something that the most wonderful person out there wants to share with someone else – the chance to have their own child! It's not a baby factory – it's simply a chance to let a much loved and wanted little one into the world.
>
> *(Michelle Evans, Submission #26)*

Much like the earlier extracts, this extract is reliant upon a set of binaries that normalize women's role as one centred upon reproduction. In this extract we see paired contrasts between 'loving and caring people' and 'moneymaking schemes', and between a 'baby factory' and 'let[ting] a much loved and wanted little one into the world'. In these contrasts the extract attends to both sides of the binary, yet makes a clear case for which side politicians should come down on. Yet in so doing, the extract takes for granted a number of assumptions, namely:

1 that surrogacy is a gift;
2 that the wellbeing in need of protection is solely children's; and
3 that surrogates are 'willing' people.

Placed together, and despite the fact that the extract speaks glowingly of surrogacy, what tends to disappear are the actual women who might act as surrogates. This is especially concerning given the only reference to an actual woman is a 'young teenage mother', precisely one of the populations of women who would be most at risk of exploitation in regards to surrogacy. Issues of exploitation and rights are more clearly (though not necessarily any less contentiously) addressed in the following extract:

> We are expecting our first child in Feb – with my sister in law acting as our surrogate. If the current legislation stays as it is we will have to wait years until we are able to adopt our own child. My sister in law will be legally recognised as the mother and her husband the father of our child even though it is not directly genetically related to them. There will be no legal recognition of our child's genetic heritage, we will have to apply for a parentage order, until that is granted we will have problems regarding accessing healthcare for our child without my sister in laws consent, should we want to travel overseas and get a passport for our child we would require my sister in laws consent. Surrogacy is about creating families; it is not about tearing mothers and babies apart like adoption. It is about giving babies back to their families.
>
> *(Ms Susan Mobbs, Submission #27)*

In this extract the personal narrative provided to a large extent overshadows some of the complexities in surrogacy by rendering salient only some of the issues. The concerns raised centre upon genetics and consent, and in so doing primarily emphasize the rights of the intended parents. Whilst it could be argued that these are circuitously aimed at supporting the child, the question must be asked as to why the parents would have concern about a member of their own family not consenting. That issues of consent are so salient seems to us to demonstrate a proprietal investment in the child, who it must be noted will always be able to access healthcare in Australia regardless of their birth certificate, and who as a child has no inherent need for a passport.

Importantly, we make these points not to argue against the personal opinions represented in the final submission included above, but rather in order to highlight the dilemmatic nature of the argument presented in this extract. In other words, if the bottom line of the submission is that surrogacy is good because it allows for the creation of families, and if altruistic surrogacy occurs in an extended family context, then what must be questioned is precisely what form of family is being invested in here. We would suggest that a possessive investment is evoked here when the concern becomes more about tangential rights than the actual fact of having a child that is desired by its family. Furthermore, there is an implicit assumption that in order to be a good woman, the woman acting as a surrogate must relinquish the child and take up an investment herself in the intended parent's possessive investment. Again, then, this is reliant upon a highly normative image of women as generous, giving and selfless child bearers who must either comply with the demands made of them, or risk being seen as causing trouble. Obviously such an image is problematic for the ways in which it limits women to tightly regulated understandings of their reproductive capacities.

Of course it must also be noted that this extract reinforces the family formation hierarchy outlined earlier, when reference is made to surrogacy being 'about creating families ... not about tearing mothers and babies apart like adoption'. Indeed, as noted earlier, the extracts that were pro-surrogacy were far from uniform in their claims, yet underpinning them was the continued emphasis upon highly gender normative roles for *all* women, not simply for women who act as surrogates. As we now discuss, this continued emphasis upon traditional roles has significant implications for the capacity of public debate to truly consider the ethics of surrogacy.

Concluding thoughts

In this chapter we presented data from three different public representations of surrogacy: media representations of heterosexual intending parents; media representations of the Baby Gammy case; and public submissions to a government inquiry. The analysis above indicates both similarities and differences in representations across the three data sets, and we discuss these differences further below.

In terms of representations of surrogacy in the mainstream media, we considered how the reproductive vulnerabilities of Australians who undertake transnational surrogacy in India are typically rendered as mere plot narratives in an overarching story of such individuals as agentic citizens who fulfil their human right to reproduction. Importantly, such representations are frequently placed alongside representations of women who act as surrogates, who are depicted as the only vulnerable people in surrogacy arrangements. This was seen in both our analysis of representations of intending parents and in our analysis of representations of the Baby Gammy case. By contrast, intending parents were able to mitigate their vulnerability through the logic of intent, as we also highlighted in relation to previous research in Chapter 1. Here, intending parents – by being represented as agentic and able to make decisions to overcome their vulnerability – are able to downplay vulnerabilities that they may otherwise face as a result of being unable to have children (Vora, 2015; Ragoné, 1994). Instead, intending parents become 'responsible' citizens who are able to make decisions, with women who act as surrogates instead assuming all vulnerability within the surrogacy arrangement.

However, narratives of agency for intending parents and vulnerability for women acting as surrogates are problematic. This is particularly due to the fact that sweeping away the reproductive vulnerabilities of those who undertake reproductive travel does nothing to either:

1 examine how such vulnerabilities are produced in social contexts that privilege genetic relatedness; or
2 conceptualize reproductive vulnerabilities as a way of thinking about what might constitute ethical reproductive travel.

By representing intending parents as overcoming vulnerability, neither of these issues can be dealt with in ways that could lead to more equal outcomes for all parties.

In terms of women acting as surrogates, it is of note that in media coverage concerning Baby Gammy, Ms Chanbua not only received specific media attention, but she was also represented in ways that can be seen as inconsistent with typical coverage whereby women who act as surrogates are seen as vulnerable but also as potentially 'bad' mothers (or indeed are not seen at all). Such representations of women acting as surrogates were commonly seen in the submission made to the inquiry into *Legislation on Altruistic Surrogacy in NSW*, where it was common to see normative representations of women, mothering and reproduction. On the other hand, while Ms Chanbua was represented as vulnerable, she was not represented as a 'bad' mother. We argue here, then, that Ms Chanbua received specific media attention because her actions in keeping Baby Gammy and not having an abortion are consistent with these normative representations of women and motherhood. This is of particular note, because the positive representations of Ms Chanbua are therefore not because she acted as a surrogate, but rather because she acted in ways consistent with normative understandings of women and motherhood.

We would also argue that acknowledging normative understandings of gender and motherhood in any discussion around surrogacy is critical to ensuring that such discussions recognize the nuanced and dilemmatic nature of arguments around surrogacy, as well as open up a space to challenge normative understandings of women and mothers. However, problematically, media representations of women involved in surrogacy arrangements rarely challenge dominant representations. Instead, there is a lack of engagement with women as autonomous beings, with there instead being a focus on women that centres normative and gendered understandings of how women are expected to behave, particularly in relation to motherhood. When such normative understandings of women and mothers are taken as a starting point for discussions of the benefits or disadvantages of surrogacy, the autonomy (or lack thereof) afforded to women acting as surrogates is rarely discussed. We would argue that a starting point for discussions concerning surrogacy ought always to be the ways in which surrogacy as a practice has the potential to either subvert or uphold women's autonomy and agency when making decisions about their bodies and reproductive capabilities.

And this is perhaps one of the most central and pressing concerns relating to critical commentary on surrogacy in the near future: how do we keep in sight both the social construction of motherhood (and thus refuse the assumption that woman = womb = mother) whilst at the same time recognizing the gendered nature of surrogacy. Furthermore, whilst it may seem redundant to state that surrogacy is gendered, what we are suggesting is that surrogacy is *normatively* gendered in that it takes the capacity of women to reproduce as a given, when in fact the very case of surrogacy occurs in most instances because some women *cannot* bear a child.

Finally, and despite concerns about how Ms Chanbua was represented, it is nonetheless notable to us that in many ways media representation of the Baby Gammy case may be construed as a turning towards the face of the Other. Admittedly, much of this turning is normative and benevolent in its understanding of Ms Chanbua's situation, but it is nonetheless of note that any recognition was accorded to her circumstances and indeed rights. Where this turning towards the Other failed, however, is in the fact that it stopped short of bringing Ms Chanbua's experiences and those of the Farnells into conversation with one another. Instead, as is typical of media coverage, they are depicted as in opposition (and perhaps they very much were in real life). A focus on how their differing vulnerabilities are similarly made intelligible in the broader contexts of globalization and capitalism would have represented a genuine intervention into how surrogacy is oriented to as a topic, and could have served to raise awareness of the problems associated with surrogacy as a response to infertility more broadly. As such, there is a critical need to open up marginalized and alternative representations concerning all people involved in surrogacy arrangements in order to provide space to really consider the impact of surrogacy on the wellbeing of those involved: issues which we take up in detail in the following chapter.

8 WAYS FORWARD

Overview

In the first chapter of this book we proposed an orientation towards surrogacy that is potentially disorienting for the ways in which it renders normative discourses and subject positions visible. By drawing attention to the capitalist logic at play in narratives and practices of surrogacy, we suggested that disorientation is an essential requirement when examining surrogacy from a critical standpoint. In this final chapter, we reflect upon the contents of this book with the aim of further 'opening up' marginalized discourses or orientations (Foucault, 2003). In doing so, our aim is not to provide guidelines as to how countries should proceed in relation to surrogacy legislation, or to dictate as to whether or not surrogacy should be viewed as acceptable by individuals. Rather, our aim is to think about how the analyses we have presented in this book demonstrate that surrogacy should remain a dis/orientation precisely so that the logics that underpin it remain firmly in our sights. We argue that when various orientations are all placed on the table together, the potential health outcomes of surrogacy can be interrogated more transparently by all parties involved, thus contributing to an acknowledgement of the operations of health (in)equity and wellbeing within the context of surrogacy arrangements. In this chapter we first provide brief summaries of the previous analytic chapters, before turning to engage with several theoretical standpoints that may help us to continue in our disorientation towards surrogacy, and thus assist us to think critically about ways forward.

The ground we have covered

In the first two chapters of this book we explored a range of theories and standpoints through which we framed the analytic chapters of this book. In particular, we outlined how the logic of capitalism offers an often under-explored and thus potentially useful framework for considering how surrogacy is constructed and enacted within current sociopolitical contexts, particularly given the potential for a focus on capitalism to be disorienting (Ahmed, 2006). In particular, we argued that focusing on the logic of capitalism and the role it plays in relation to surrogacy could encourage a focus on the gendered norms that surround surrogacy arrangements. In making some of those norms and discourses visible, our aim was to interrogate the subject positions and identities available to people involved in surrogacy, and in this final chapter we explore the health implications of those subject positions. In particular, we draw on Foucault to explore how we can 'open up' marginalized discourses to create more equitable discussions of health for all involved. We argue that opening up marginalized discourses and interrogating available identities is an important part of creating an ethical stance to surrogacy that allows us to explore the differential effects of power and status (Stainton Rogers, 1991).

In Chapter 3 we considered data pertaining to women who act as surrogates in order to consider the various orientations to surrogacy displayed by these differing groups of women – at least in relation to representations of them in surrogacy advertisements and documentary projects. In both this chapter and Chapter 4 we explored the competing discourse of love or money, and the identities that these discourses make available to both women who act as surrogates, and intending parents. Specifically in Chapter 3, we highlighted how women who act as surrogates are positioned as vulnerable, and how they are required to represent themselves in ways that align them with particular cultural values and norms which differ depending on the sociocultural context in which they live and work. As we consider further in this final chapter of the book, it is important to examine the potential implications of such a requirement, and the potential health and wellbeing outcomes that follow for women who act as surrogates.

In Chapter 4 we turned from women who act as surrogates, to consider the orientations that intending parents display towards surrogacy arrangements within their advertisements. Our analysis suggested that intending parents frequently display complex orientations to the binary of love or money, as also noted in relation to women who act as surrogates. Specifically, we suggested that intending parents frequently claim that women who act as surrogates should do so out of altruism rather than a desire for money, yet that at the same time the payment of money allows intending parents to 'contract out' of any relationship with the woman carrying their child. In turn, we suggested that the 'contracting out' of relationships with women who act as surrogates allows intending parents to claim the pregnancy as their own. Specifically, we suggested that certain normative constructions of surrogacy allow intending parents to minimize the vulnerability inherent in their position as a result of being unable to reproduce through heterosex. This minimization is a result of both claims to agency (i.e. the intent to have children), as well as their location within capitalist contexts which allow intending parents to remove women who act as surrogates from the picture and thus justify their position as parents. In essence, we argued that vulnerability is shifted from intending parents to women who act as surrogates. Interestingly, and as we argue further below, both the vulnerability of women who act as surrogates and the shifting of vulnerability of intending parents are likely to have deleterious effects on health.

Having considered both women who act as surrogates and intending parents, in Chapter 5 we explored how storybook representations of children born through surrogacy arrangements place an injunction upon such children to display a particular orientation towards their conception, gestation and birth. In exploring storybooks written for children who were conceived via surrogacy arrangements, we outlined how these books reinforce the importance of the norm of genetic relatedness – and how this works to reproduce an idea that it is only *some* children who are priceless by suggesting that children who are genetically related to the parent/s raising them are seen as more desirable than children who are not. Such an understanding means that children who are not genetically related to their parents – such as children in foster care or adoption – are seen as less desirable, expanding on the points we made in this regard in Chapter 2. We also explored gendered norms seen in terms of women and their role in having babies, and the formative role this plays with regard to sociocultural representations of women. Following Wendy Stainton Rogers' (1991) critical health approach to understanding cultural norms and their impact on health, we argued that the wellbeing of children born through surrogacy may be impacted by norms concerning the differential value accorded to children.

In Chapter 6 we considered surrogacy clinic websites, and the ways in which they market to gay intending parents. Here, we saw that clinics situate gay men within a logic of reproductive citizenship and capitalism, where genetic relatedness is again privileged. In order to replicate these norms, however, women who act as surrogates are rendered invisible on the websites via the naturalization of their bodies as solely purposed for having children and giving birth. Our analysis in Chapter 6 suggested not only that the websites failed to engage with the potential vulnerability of women who act as surrogates, but that the websites also fail to acknowledge the potential vulnerabilities experienced by intending parents. As noted above, this failure is likely to have ongoing impacts on the health of all those involved in surrogacy arrangements, and again we explore this further below.

Finally, in Chapter 7 we explored public representations of surrogacy in relation to a variety of media and other public sources. In this chapter, we explored how discourses of vulnerability and intentionality differentially affect intending parents and women who act as surrogates, such that women who act as surrogates are represented as vulnerable while intending parents are represented as agentic – echoing our findings throughout the book. In addition, we explored how public representations of surrogacy draw upon normative accounts of women to argue either for or against surrogacy arrangements. Given the relationship of the media to the health and wellbeing of those represented within in it (i.e. the media can open up or close down attention to particular health inequalities), it is likely that these representations impact on the health of the people represented within public discourse, perhaps particularly by providing individuals with a narrow set of subject positions through which they may be rendered intelligible (Foucault, 2003; Riggs, 2005; Blackman & Walkerdine, 2001). In the remainder of this chapter, then, we explore several frameworks that may help us to further consider how to think about surrogacy in the future, before bringing all of these considerations back to an understanding of health.

Seriality

In his *Critique of Dialectical Reason* (1976), Sartre introduced the idea of 'seriality'; namely, the conceptualization of a group of people who are passively connected as a result of their shared practices, goals and habits rather than joined through active group membership, essential characteristics or external norms. Within the concept of seriality, 'series' concern flexible groups of people who are considered as joined by shared orientations (e.g. standing in line for a bus). As such, seriality provides a framework for thinking about how individuals within any particular series may reflexively enact a particular norm themselves. In this sense, then, seriality focuses on the imposition of *a group norm about the group*, in contrast to Gramsci's account of hegemony, where an external norm is first imposed, and then taken up by, any given group (Eagleton, 1991).

In discussing 'fertility tourists' in the United Kingdom, Nicky Hudson and Lorraine Culley (2011) draw upon the concept of seriality, arguing that it was developed as a response to the ways in which individuals relate to capitalism and consumption, and therefore provides a 'useful means of thinking about the relationship between social structures and the individual' (Hudson & Culley, 2011, p. 574). Specifically, by breaking down higher order categories of groups of people, Hudson and Culley argue that the concept of seriality allows us to explore individual or subgroup differences within larger groups who are generally classed together according to the existing structures in any given sociocultural or political context. For example, social scientists have used the concept of seriality to critique the assumption that those belonging to a particular group will necessarily experience similar identities or share essential characteristics (Young, 1994).

Hudson and Culley (2011) note that the critique of group norms and assumptions about cohesive group membership as developed within the concept of seriality has been particularly applied in relation to gender and class. They further note that it cannot actually be assumed that all within a group necessarily share common characteristics beyond higher-order ones such as being a woman or being accorded a lower socioeconomic status. Scholars such as Iris Marion Young (1994) have used seriality as a framework through which to think about group membership – such as being a woman – as produced by society rather than reflecting innate characteristics which group people within a given series together. The concept of seriality, then, gives us a framework through which to explore more closely passive membership and its implications for individuals. Specifically, as Hudson and Culley (2011) note:

> In this model, 'series' are differentiated from more formal 'groups' by virtue of their passive membership. Whereas a group (according to Sartre) is a collection of people who identify with one another, recognize their common group membership and are united by common goals and actions, a series may contain individuals who are only passively unified around common objects and who are engaged in pursuing their own individual ends. A key issue here is that individuals can be simultaneously and loosely associated with a number of series (women, employees, treatment seekers, etc.), without needing to actively identify as a group in an ongoing, conscious and essentialist manner.
>
> *(p. 574)*

As such, the concept of seriality – and series rather than purposive groups – provides a useful way in which to think about the series of people we have explored within this book. Importantly, by considering people as series we do not claim that any of the parties involved in surrogacy that we have focused on within this book are necessarily purposive collectives who share essential characteristics that bring them together, or that we can ascribe characteristics of one member to all others. Rather, we argue here that various people involved in surrogacy become grouped as a series by the fact that it appears that they frequently and uncritically adopt within-group norms, thus meaning that we see similar discourses drawn upon by the diverse series of people situated within the context of surrogacy, even if in differing ways across contexts (for example, the binary of love or money, or narratives about what constitutes 'nature'). In relation to fertility travellers, Hudson and Culley (2011) suggest that:

> In the case of the present fertility travellers, the objects and practices that unified the participants were related to their access to resources, both financial and cultural, their engagement with bio-technology, their pursuit of parenthood and the agency that they enacted in order to achieve this goal. It may be argued that those who travel overseas also form part of a wider series that is fertility treatment seekers. This larger generic collectivity is also united passively around these objects and practices.
>
> *(p. 578)*

Using this conceptualization of the series, we can see how people involved in various aspects of surrogacy can also be seen as a series. In the case of intending parents, many of the points discussed by Hudson and Culley above in relation to fertility travellers pertain to intending parents as a series, including access to financial and cultural resources, pursuit of (in many cases desired genetic) parenthood, and claims to agency. Moreover, intending parents can be seen as a series as a result of their shared experiences concerning challenges with reproduction. Importantly, by seeking surrogacy arrangements as a way to minimize vulnerability, and by often being complicit with a system that reduces the bodies of women acting as surrogates to objects serving a purpose, the series of intending parents can also be seen as uncritically accepting a set of social norms and structures which reproduce existing power relations.

The concept of series also offers useful ways to think about women who act as surrogates – particularly given that viewing them as a group essentializes largely heterogeneous experiences that differ widely depending on the social and political context in which women live and the circumstances that lead to them acting as surrogates. Conversely, however, considering women who act as surrogates as part of a series rather than a group takes into account some aspects of the shared circumstances that lead certain women to act as surrogates, whilst being mindful of their diverse social conditions. As such, the shared characteristics that unite women who act as surrogates may be less obvious, and is likely to vary according to social contexts – as we saw in Chapter 3. However, potential practices which unite women who act as surrogates as a series include a set of norms which construct women's bodies as reducible to objects that can produce good (i.e. children), a presumed orientation to either 'love or money' which prompts them to engage in surrogacy, a shared (although highly heterogeneous) social situation which positions surrogacy as a viable option to provide income (in the case of compensated or commercial surrogacy), and shared experiences of social positioning which requires particular normative behaviours predicated upon compliance.

More broadly, considering all parties involved in surrogacy as series rather than groups also provides us with a position from which to critique the logic of capitalism that otherwise seeks to present each group of people in ways which accord with the production of capital and goods. Given the flexibility of series and the way in which the framework of seriality allows us to take into account social and political contexts, series provide us with a position from which to see how people involved in surrogacy arrangements are responding to normative social conditions, rather than as a product of essentialist characteristics that group them together by virtue of their similarity. For example, many of the representations of – or orientations towards – surrogacy explored in this book revolve around issues related to capitalism. For example: the orientations of intending parents focus on norms of genetic relatedness and priceless children, both of which arguably can be traced back to capitalism; the orientations of women acting as surrogates reflect a capitalist logic which positions their bodies as objects capable of producing goods; and so on. As such, combining people together based on their position within surrogacy and assuming that they are a group sharing essential criteria and a shared identity elides the broader social contexts and the differences between these contexts which actually lead them to engage in surrogacy arrangements.

Seriality, then, offers us a useful framework with which to critique essentialism in surrogacy. Indeed, we argue that seriality can be seen as a tool for reading for disorientation when considering those involved in surrogacy arrangements. For example, by being forced to forgo the comfortable language of the group, we are required to look at how a series is produced through inter- and within-group norms, as well as the ways in which people can move in and out of particular subject positions. As seen above, interrogating particular norms or sets of social circumstances calls into question many of the normative assumptions involved in surrogacy, including particular identities commonly assumed to be constitutive of universal, within-group norms. In exploring how members of a series are constructed as sharing particular trait (e.g. agency in the case of intending parents, a desire to help in the case of women acting as surrogates, and so on), we can see how particularly dominant constructions of identity come to represent all members of a series and define their identity, thereby constructing surrogacy itself in particular ways (e.g. through a capitalist framework which positions some people as agentic consumers and others as passive producers of goods).

Moreover, Sartre's concept of series is highly flexible, in that people can move in and out of membership – thereby disorienting considerations of groups as involving fixed and stable traits. Unlike groups considered to be inflexible (e.g. you either are a woman or you aren't), series allow people to take up identities related to the series and put them down again as social, cultural and individual situations change. Again, this aspect of seriality offers us a useful standpoint from which to investigate the capitalist orientation that we have argued shapes surrogacy practices, in that it allows us to focus on specific discursive framings rather than assumed-to-be homogenous groups. Focusing on groups as flexible series rather than as immutable is important for the capacity it provides us to consider sociocultural situations and their effects on people. And just as importantly, and following the work of Halberstam (2005), we might argue that focusing on series rather than groups offers us one entry point into disorienting capitalism itself: by understanding the current iterations of the 'surrogacy series' as a product of capitalism, we might consider, for example, other ways in which reproduction and parenthood might be understood (such as with regard to Ragoné's (1994) early work on genetic surrogacy, or Teman's (2010) work on how surrogacy operates in Israel). This is not to suggest that surrogacy might function entirely outside of the capitalist market, but rather that surrogacy as a series is not wholly limited to a capitalist imaginary.

Finally, the flexibility to move in and out of series has important implications for health and wellbeing. In particular, the concept of the series allows us to explore how people involved in each series may be differentially affected by surrogacy arrangements. As such, a woman acting as a surrogate in India cannot be assumed to be likely to experience the same health outcomes as a woman acting as a surrogate in a country in the West. In addition, considering people involved in surrogacy in relation to Sartre's idea of the series also facilitates the movement of people in and out of series, allowing them to take up and put down specific subject positions rather than always inhabiting them in a fixed or essentialist way; a fact which again has implications for health and health equity, as we shall see in the following section.

Capitalism, vulnerability and alternative discourses

At the beginning of this book we introduced capitalism as a structuring logic through which surrogacy is made intelligible, and in so doing we sought to orient ourselves explicitly towards capitalism when considering the various aspects of surrogacy that we explored throughout the book. We sought to orient ourselves to capitalism given that we argued that this orientation was in fact a dominant logic through which surrogacy is rendered intelligible, and therefore – following Sara Ahmed (2006) – this orientation is typically invisible or unmarked. However, in orienting to capitalism we also sought to orient ourselves *away* from capitalism (Halberstam, 2005). In particular – by unpacking how capitalism frames both the desire to have genetically related children (and surrogacy as one mode of achieving this) – our aim has been to create space for the possibility of alternative discourses and ways of understanding surrogacy for all involved.

In Chapter 2 we introduced health equity through the work of Wendy Stainton Rogers (1991), and her call to use cultural critique as a way of understanding constructions of health. We noted that any considerations of surrogacy must be concerned with the differential effects of power and status upon all parties involved in surrogacy arrangements, including the ways in which individuals are rendered vulnerable within both cultural contexts where reproductivity is privileged, and where the practice of surrogacy is normalized. Such an approach to surrogacy and health is clearly consistent with the tenets of critical health approaches to health equity. In the sections that follow, we consider how to move forward in our discussions of surrogacy and health in ways which foreground the health of all people involved in surrogacy arrangements. As discussed above, we will also draw upon Sartre's concept of seriality to provide a framework from which to consider the health of all parties involved in surrogacy, while also critiquing the idea that people involved in surrogacy can be considered cohesive groups for whom similar health considerations are required.

First, it is important to revisit the concept of vulnerability, a central theme running through nearly all the chapters in this book as we have considered the various aspects of surrogacy. Specifically, we have argued that a capitalist logic renders us all vulnerable to the operations of the state and the imperative to be producers or consumers of goods – although vulnerability is accorded differentially to different parties involved in surrogacy. In terms of this relationship between capitalism and vulnerability, Halberstam (2005) argues:

> If we destabilize the meaning of capitalism using poststructuralist critiques of identity and signification, then we can begin to see the multiplicity of non-capitalist forms that constitute, supplement, and abridge global capitalism, but we can also begin to imagine, by beginning to see, the alternatives to capitalism that already exist and are presently under construction. Gibson-Graham calls for the 'querying' of globalization through a wide-ranging recognition of its incomplete status, its discontinuities, instabilities, and vulnerabilities.
>
> *(p. 12)*

Here, following Jack Halberstam, we argue that capitalism produces vulnerability via the drive to produce (and specifically *re*produce) that we have explored throughout this book in relation to reproductive vulnerabilities. Specifically, in the case of intending parents, we have argued that reproductive vulnerability – including a focus on the privileging of genetic relationships – leads to intending parents participating in surrogacy arrangements in the first place. Importantly, however, this vulnerability is seen as effectively passed on to women who act as surrogates when intending parents draw upon the notion of 'intent' to overcome individual vulnerability, with potential health implications discussed below. In the case of women who act as surrogates, we have highlighted how women are seen as vulnerable as a result of their social positioning and the potential for exploitation and commodification potentially inherent in surrogacy arrangements when viewed through the lens of capitalism. In this section we return to the concept of vulnerability in terms of all parties, and in so doing potentially contribute to the destabilization of capitalism itself by highlighting how it too is vulnerable. Moreover, we suggest that by considering all parties involved in surrogacy as a series, we can open up dialogues concerning individual wellbeing, which in turn allows us to see those 'potential alternatives to capitalism that already exist and are presently under construction' proposed by Halberstam.

In a sense, then, orienting to capitalism in order to destabilize it provides us with one way in which we can think about surrogacy going forward, particularly in relation to considerations of health. Capitalism, as we have seen throughout this book, can lead to a situation in which only specific parties involved in surrogacy are considered in relation to health – and even then only very narrowly. For example, Raywat Deonandan and colleagues (2012) suggest in relation to surrogacy, when it is arranged through clinics, that:

> The clinic receives payment from one party (the client) and performs a procedure on a second party (the surrogate). In other words, one entity represents both the paying client and the paid surrogate. Several stakeholders, with potentially competing interests, are at play: the client, her spouse, the surrogate and, of course, the child resulting from the process. The potential is great for conflicts of interest, especially when clinical decisions must be made that weigh monetary cost against the health of the surrogate. In such scenarios, the cynic would suspect that the interests of the paying client will prevail, even to the detriment of the health of the surrogate. At the very least, the incentive for such favouritism is financial, whereas the sole disincentive is moral.
>
> *(p. 3)*

This situation represents clearly the way in which a capitalist logic can lead to differential health – and ethical – outcomes for those involved, whereby those who can pay will always receive better treatment. Correspondingly, they suggest, 'the ethics at play are business ethics, not medical ethics' (p. 3) – and taken further, we would suggest that this is in fact a normative ethics under capitalism.

Moving forward, Deonandan and colleagues (2012) note that: 'As the global reproductive travel industry expands, it is incumbent upon all parties, government and civil society included, to explore options for mitigating the many ethical challenges with which the phenomenon presents us' (p. 745). We would argue that this is true, but also we would also argue for more. In orienting to capitalism, we can see how differential health outcomes impact the health of those involved in surrogacy as a result of a primary focus on labour and goods. However, as we noted earlier, and again following Halberstam (2005), in orienting to capitalism we must also ultimately aim to orient *away* from it. We would suggest here that an orientation away from capitalism involves 'opening up' marginalized or alternative discourses which do not simplistically endorse the status quo of privileging certain modes of reproduction or certain people on the basis of their access to capital (Foucault, 2003). One way in which we can do this is by considering all parties involved in surrogacy arrangements as members of series rather than groups, so that we can emphasize both their individuality, and (perhaps more importantly) the social, cultural and political situations in which they find themselves and which lead them to engage in a surrogacy arrangement. In considering people as belonging to series in this way, we can ensure that broader societal drives to reproduce are interrogated for their specific health and wellbeing impacts on those involved in surrogacy arrangements.

Another way we can open up alternative discourses is by considering the operations of power in the drive to reproduce. In *Society Must be Defended*, Foucault (2003) outlines the role of state power in relation to race (as an essentialized category). Specifically, he considers how state power is deployed to position people in categories as either 'good' or 'bad', 'superior' or 'inferior', and so on. By drawing on essentialist categories in this way, it becomes easier for the state to control populations: with control and power in this sense being closely related to discourse. Indeed, as Vivien Burr (1995) argues in relation to Foucault's theorization of power, discourse and power are intricately bound together in that power is an effect of discourse through which people are able to define the world and others, thereby producing and reinforcing particular claims to 'knowledge' or truth. Furthermore, by functioning as what Foucault termed a 'technology of subjectification', public representations such as those seen in the media (and discussed in Chapter 7) play a central role in constituting people as subjects through the ways in which a limited range of subject positions are made intelligible (Blackman & Walkerdine, 2001).

In relation to surrogacy, then, it becomes clear that positioning individuals as workers in the cogs of capitalism – and particularly through reproductive vulnerability – allows the state to control populations in ways that reinforce specific forms of normative family structures and gendered behaviours. We have seen this throughout the chapters of this book when we have addressed the drive to have genetically related children in order to ensure that family structures adhere to those suited to the needs of the state: specifically families working to raise the next generation of compliant workers. One way to address this, then, is to examine what drives the desire for genetically related children, and to then be able to consider how that drive potentially prevents some individuals from considering other options for starting a family (such as foster care or adoption), or from considering the broader ramifications of the decision to engage in reproductive travel (which has broad ranging ethical reproductions, as we explore in more detail below). Opening up alternative discourses, then, could include a deconstruction of normative understandings of kinship, as well as critique of the drive to maintain population levels in the West by having genetically related children rather than by considering the role of immigration in a world where population levels are already high.

To return to intending parents in the context of surrogacy arrangements, vulnerability is therefore always already present as a result of their inability to reproduce via heterosex. However, we have argued that the vulnerability of intending parents is minimized within a capitalist logic, which places intending parents as the agentic party within the surrogacy arrangement; they become able to act out their drive to be 'good' citizens by having genetically related children born through surrogacy arrangements. Nevertheless, the reproductive vulnerability that we introduced at the beginning of this book remains, and likely has insidious effects on health and wellbeing – including in relation to the impact of shame on overall health. As we have argued elsewhere (Riggs & Due, 2012), shame frequently accompanies infertility, and as such, a focus on shame is important, for to focus on shame is to focus on vulnerability. Again, one way in which intending parents potentially reduce fertility-related shame is to become the agentic party in a surrogacy arrangement – with their intent represented as the reason a child was born; a representation which positions intending parents as fulfilling their obligation to the state to have children by virtue of their intent.

Finally with regard to vulnerability, and as we noted above, it is vital that we examine how surrogacy provides us with an example of how capitalism itself is vulnerable. A simple example of this appears in the science of reproduction itself. As we know from 'success' rates of IVF since its beginnings, very little has changed, despite the considerable growth in the use of this technology. As such, given that capitalism is reliant upon the production of a workforce and a consuming class (and their intersections), this reliance is always already tentative, given the increased rates at which many people delay reproduction, the attendant impact of this upon fertility, and thus the increased reliance upon reproductive technologies. This is not to say that the world population is not growing at an exponential rate, but rather to highlight the contingency and vulnerability of reproduction within capitalist societies. Another example of the vulnerability of capitalism appears in the work of Sharmila Rudrappa (2015), who deftly explores the intersections of the garment industry and the surrogacy industry in India. Since the time that Rudrappa collected her data, surrogacy in India has been closed to foreign nationals, meaning that as a source of reproductive labour, India (and many other countries that have followed suit) is no longer available as a resource for Western capitalist societies. Again, none of this is to suggest that capitalism is still not a powerful force to be reckoned with: we have demonstrated throughout this book that it very much is. Rather, it is to suggest that capitalism is nonetheless vulnerable, to the circulation of workers, its capacity to produce goods and the variabilities of the market.

Surrogacy and health

In the previous section we explored how opening up alternative discourses concerning surrogacy has the potential to assist in thinking about ways forward. When normative understandings of women and mothers remain the primary target of any commentary on surrogacy (either for or against surrogacy arrangements), what disappears are both the actual disparities that result in certain groups of women acting as surrogates, and other groups of people making use of surrogacy services, as well as any sort of productive commentary on what practices and policies would need to be in place for surrogacy to be a truly ethical practice that refuses normative discourses of motherhood and their attendant practices of commodification. As such, we turn here to explore some of these health implications.

Throughout this book thus far we have discussed how intending parents are rendered vulnerable as a result of their challenges concerning reproduction. We have shown how there is an attempt to pass this vulnerability on to women acting as surrogates; or at least to overcome it through agency and intent when undertaking surrogacy. However, we would nonetheless argue that in fact this attempt to overcome vulnerability ignores a range of very real vulnerabilities associated with reproduction – many of which some intending parents will have experienced. These include events such as pregnancy loss, grief associated with attempting to have a child and being unable to achieve or maintain a pregnancy, health issues which lead to infertility, and so forth. All of these challenges are likely to have health and wellbeing implications for intending parents. In attempting to overlook this vulnerability we suggest that there is a shift away from health for intending parents and onto an individualist, neoliberal outlook which emphasizes the way in which individuals can overcome health challenges; a problematic assumption, particularly when the way in which those challenges are overcome poses real risks to the health of others – as we discuss below in relation to women who act as surrogates. Thus, as Marilyn Strathern (1992) suggests: 'new techniques of "fertilisation" do not remedy fertility as such, but childlessness; they enable a potential parent to have access to the fertility of others' (p. 37). What remains, then, is vulnerability to the injunction to reproductivity as a taken for granted norm (i.e. something that can be achieved without 'assistance'), which the fact of having children does not per se remedy.

Vulnerability and its impact on health can also been seen in relation to children born through surrogacy arrangements. For example, as we saw in Chapter 5, while research shows that the mental and physical health of children born through surrogacy is on a par with that of children conceived in other ways, some practices related to surrogacy remain which may render them vulnerable. In particular, this includes structural practices such as the prohibition on contact with the woman who carried them (as is the case in India), and some instances where the information about their egg donor (if there was one) is not recorded. Of course, throughout this book we have critiqued the privileging of genetic relatedness over other forms of kinship. Nevertheless, knowing genetic information can be important for health reasons, and it is thus worth mentioning that the *inability* to know all those involved in their conception, gestation and birth may be considered to have potentially negative long-term consequences for children conceived via surrogacy arrangements, and thus vulnerabilities in the broader context of societies that privilege both genetic relatedness along with one's ability or indeed right to have contact with those to whom one is genetically related.

In relation to women who act as surrogates, we suggest that the lack of control potentially experienced by women may have implications for their health, particularly given findings from previous research concerning the impact of lack of control on health outcomes (e.g. Fisher & Baum, 2010). For example, whereas intending parents are seen as having agency which they use to overcome vulnerability through claims to intent (even if such intent is only a construct produced by capitalism), women who act as surrogates are generally required to occupy subject positions in which they are compliant, humble and prepared to act in accordance with the wishes of intending parents. If these requirements translate from our analysis of advertisements and documentaries into real-world actions (and we would suggest that they do, given previous research by Vora, 2009, and Pande, 2011), then we argue that this onus placed on women who act as surrogates is likely to have long-term implications for health – and particularly for health equity – for this group of women. Indeed, the requirement for women who act as surrogates to be seen as compliant producers of goods has the potential to undermine women as individuals, and further compound negative impacts on health and wellbeing.

More traditional health outcomes also need to be considered in relation to women who act as surrogates. As we have seen, the construction of women who act as surrogates as goods producing a product often means that their bodies are subject to strict regimes and control during the pregnancy. In the Indian context, this has typically meant that they live in dormitory-like accommodation and are closely monitored. It is notable, though, that India has one of the highest maternal and pregnancy-related mortality rates in the world outside the context of surrogacy (Bailey, 2011). These deaths are generally related to the sociocultural context in which women live, including poverty, lack of education and social status, and accordingly Bailey argues that: 'if the demographic of women signing up for surrogacy work overlaps significantly with the demographic of women who are medically vulnerable, then these injustices must be part of the conversation' (p. 731). Many women who act as surrogates may have experienced poor health prior to their surrogacy pregnancy, and may well experience poor health again after they have given birth and return to their families and homes. In some instances, the surrogate pregnancy may exacerbate these – such as when women are required to have a caesarean to deliver the baby (Johnson, Blyth & Hammarberg, 2014).

While the same specific set of social situations are not faced by women in higher income countries who act as surrogates, it is often true that women acting as surrogates in compensated or commercial surrogacy arrangements are from lower socioeconomic groups regardless of the country in which they live, and may face similar – if not quite as extreme – situations. For example, Alison Bailey (2011) argues that it may be likely that women in the West who act as surrogates are also women who have limited or no access to healthcare, and who may consider acting as a surrogate in order to compensate for income which they would otherwise be unable to achieve. As in India or Thailand, women in the West may also be able to access better healthcare while they act as a surrogate than they can at other times. Following on from this differential access to healthcare, then, Bailey argues that:

> Maternal health is a human right. When reproductive health care is more accessible to women during their contract pregnancies than it is for women during their own pregnancies, then surrogacy workers have more reproductive rights when they are birthing for others than they do while having their own families.
>
> *(p. 734)*

When we consider this through the logic of capitalism and its impact on women who act as surrogates, then, it becomes clear that capitalism on its own will not provide sufficient care for women outside of their surrogacy pregnancies. Indeed, capitalism on its own clearly does not lead to adequate maternal health for all women. Moreover, some authors (e.g. Deonandan et al., 2012; Ressler, Jaeger & Lindheim, 2012) have suggested that in the context of surrogacy, care is typically limited to strictly those elements that will lead to a healthy pregnancy, and do not extend to other aspects of care such as mental health concerns related to pregnancy or other health concerns which will not impact the baby. Again, this is unsurprising when we focus on capitalism, since the logic of capitalism would suggest that clients are expected to pay only for those services which lead to the goods which they are paying for. Clearly, then, the workings of capitalism in relation to surrogacy highlight problematic health and health equity outcomes.

Transnational surrogacy in low- and middle-income countries also has health equity impacts more broadly. For example, Andrea Whittaker (2011) notes that richer clients travelling internationally often require more resources than clients living in the country themselves (Whittaker suggest up to four or five times in the case of Thailand), and that transnational patients in private hospitals has led to a 'brain drain' from public hospitals. Moreover, Whittaker suggests that there is little crossover of services or resources, meaning that transnational surrogacy services do not generally lead to improvements in healthcare or maternity services elsewhere within the health system in a country, despite this logic often being used as a justification for capitalist and neoliberal approaches to fertility travel. Instead, the capitalist logic underlying many surrogacy arrangements may in fact simply result in a system of supply and demand for those who can pay, and will not lead to benefits for all, but rather sustain localized services for those with means.

Again, the potentially negative impact that surrogacy has in low- and middle-income countries highlights the importance of explicitly orienting to capitalism when considering surrogacy. That is, dominant representations of surrogacy typically represent surrogacy industries through representations of poor or 'lower status' women for whom surrogacy may bring an income. Consequently, the only image of vulnerability we see within representations of surrogacy is one of relatively poor women choosing to act as surrogates and their families, and the accompanying 'generosity' of surrogacy clinics and intending parents in 'helping' women move out of poverty. Here, then, alternative discourses which could assist in relation to health would be those which consider the contribution that high-income countries ought to make when their citizens travel for reproductive services such as surrogacy (similar to arguments that have been made in the context of transnational adoption, see Riggs, 2009).

As we noted in the first chapter of this book, a critical approach to surrogacy, then, moves beyond surrogacy as simply a mode of reproduction. Instead, we have argued that a critical health approach to surrogacy considers the role of state power and norms, particularly in relation to the capitalist logic which underlies the workings of the state and which produces those norms. In orienting to surrogacy in this way, we can see how surrogacy is framed by a capitalist marketplace in which the focus is not on the health and wellbeing of individual humans on their own terms. Instead, 'health' is framed by the ways in which individuals can contribute to the health of the capitalist state by reproducing – with some people seen as agentic subjects in this interchange (e.g. intending parents) and others as passive objects producing goods (e.g. women acting as surrogates). However, when viewed this way, all parties involved in surrogacy can be seen as cogs in the wider machinery of capitalism, in which only very specific health interventions are provided in order to produce healthy babies, a situation which leads to large health inequities and does little to challenges structures which produce those inequalities.

Others (e.g. Markens, 2007; Whittaker, 2014) have suggested that, in order to move forward, there needs to be more of a focus on an underlying ethics in relation to surrogacy. Such a discussion would move beyond the individual rights of those involved in surrogacy to instead consider an overarching ethics that does not lead to competing rights discourses (e.g. the right to have a child versus the right to proper compensation). One response to this is suggested by Vora (2009), who highlights the potential for women who act as surrogates in India to be woven into the kinship narratives of intending parents and their families through a sense of duty. This sense of duty, Kalindi Vora suggests, is one that typically informs Indian families, and is something that could be taken up by intended parents when they engage in transnational surrogacy. Obviously claims to kinship with Indian women hold the potential to be taken up in benevolent ways by intending parents, or in ways that function disingenuously to feign kinship when really it is not desired. But recognizing that intended parents are always already in a dependent relationship to women who act as surrogates (rather than simply treating women who act as surrogates as 'wombs for hire' who are expected to disappear after the birth of child) may go at least some way towards encouraging recognition of the global context in which transnational surrogacy occurs, one in which dominant discourses of family and consumerism produce vulnerabilities that impact upon all people, albeit differentially.

We are of course not suggesting that having an ongoing relationship with women who act as surrogates ameliorates the hardships women who act as surrogates face, nor the ways in which the surrogacy industry commodifies their bodies. But at the very least, recognizing the relationships between those in the higher-income countries and those in low- to middle-income countries may encourage greater understanding amongst the former as to the complex interdependencies between the two cultural contexts, both in terms of the differences between the contexts (where one group stand to benefit at the expense of another), and the similarities (where the global market positions us all as vulnerable citizens). Focusing on vulnerability – turning towards the face of the Other – is thus one step towards enacting ways of achieving one's desires that do not require treating another as an object for consumption, for to do so, following Levinas, would be to treat oneself as an object in turn (Levinas & Kearney, 1986). Instead, accepting and speaking of vulnerability requires recognition of the damaging and dangerous logic that underpins the global marketplace, and a willingness to refuse to unthinkingly take up a place within this logic as a way of denying our own vulnerability.

Moving forward, then, it is important to imagine a future in which the health and wellbeing of all individuals who are currently involved in surrogacy arrangements can be foregrounded within broader sociocultural contexts which take into account potential health disparities and health (in)equities. Indeed, it is important to imagine a future in which the health and wellbeing of people is considered even *before* they engage in surrogacy arrangements. If we move beyond capitalist approaches to surrogacy which prioritize the exchange of goods and labour – and indeed which position babies as goods in the first place – then we can begin to see how health equity requires specific responses to individual reproductive desires. Such responses would situate individuals as series within a broader global context within which the ethics of surrogacy arrangements must be located, and which may potentially involve not engaging with the surrogacy industry, given its enmeshment with the machinations of capitalism.

REFERENCES

ABC News. (2016). Baby Gammy: Surrogacy row family cleared of abandoning child with Down syndrome in Thailand. 14 April. Retrieved 18 May 2016, from www.abc.net.au/news/2016–04–14/baby-gammy-twin-must-remain-with-family-wa-court-rules/7326196.

Ahmed, S. (2004). Declarations of whiteness: The non-performativity of anti-racism. *Borderlands*, *3*(2). Retrieved 8 April 2016, from www.borderlands.net.au/vol. 3no2_2004/ahmed_declarations.htm.

Ahmed, S. (2006). *Queer phenomenology: Orientations, objects, others*. Durham, NC: Duke University Press.

Allen, A. L. (1990). Surrogacy, slavery, and the ownership of life. *Harvard Journal of Law and Public Policy, 13*, 139–149.

Appleby, J. B. & Karnein, A. J. (2014). On the moral importance of genetic ties in families. In T. Freeman, S. Graham, F. Ebtehaj & M. Richards (Eds), *Relatedness in assisted reproduction: Families, origins and identities* (pp. 79–97). Cambridge: Cambridge University Press.

Ariès, P. (1962). *Centuries of childhood: A social history of family life*. Trans. R. Baldick. New York: Alfred A. Knopf.

Atkins, P. J. (2005). Fattening children or fattening farmers? School milk in Britain, 1921–1941. *The Economic History Review*, *58*(1), 57–78.

Bailey, A. (2011). Reconceiving surrogacy: Toward a reproductive justice account of Indian surrogacy. *Hypatia*, *26*(4), 715–741.

Barlass, T. (2011). 'Look at Mia. How can this be a crime?' asks mother. *The Age*, 23 January, p. 3.

Baslington, H. (2002). The social organization of surrogacy: Relinquishing a baby and the role of payment in the psychological detachment process. *Journal of Health Psychology*, 7, 57–71.

Becker, G., Butler, A. & Nachtigall, R. D. (2005). Resemblance talk: A challenge for parents whose children were conceived with donor gametes in the US. *Social Science and Medicine*, *61*(6), 1300–1309.

Berend, Z. (2016). 'We are all carrying someone else's child': Relatedness and relationships in third-party reproduction. *American Anthropologist*, *118*, 24–36.

Berkowitz, D. & Marsiglio, W. (2007). Gay men: Negotiating procreative, father, and family identities. *Journal of Marriage and Family*, *69*(2), 366–381.

Billig, M. (1999). Whose claims? Whose ordinariness? Rhetoric and ideology in conversation analysis. *Discourse and Society*, *10*(4), 543–547.

Blackman, L. & Walkerdine, V. (2001). *Mass hysteria: Critical psychology and media studies.* Hampshire: Palgrave.

Blake, L., Zadeh, S., Statham, H. & Freeman, T. (2014). Families created by assisted reproduction: Children's perspectives. In T. Freeman, S. Graham, F. Ebtehaj & M. Richards (Eds), *Relatedness in assisted reproduction: Families, origins, identities* (pp. 251–269). Cambridge: Cambridge University Press.

Blyth, E. (2008). Cross border reproductive services. International Federation of Social Workers. Retrieved 17 September 2012, from http://ifsw.org/policies/cross-border-reproductive-services/

Bridgewater, P. D. (2001). Un/re/dis covering slave breeding in thirteenth amendment jurisprudence. *Washington and Lee Race and Ethnic Ancestry Law Journal*, 7, 11–43.

Burr, V. (1995). *An introduction to social constructionism.* London: Routledge.

Butler, J. (2004). *Precarious life: The power of mourning and violence.* London: Verso.

Calvo, E. (2008). 'Most farmers prefer blondes': The dynamics of anthroparchy in animals' becoming meat. *Journal for Critical Animal Studies*, *6*(1), 32–45.

Celcer, I. (2014). *Hope and Will have a baby: The gift of surrogacy.* New York: Graphite Press.

Clarke, A. E. (1998). *Disciplining reproduction: Modernity, American life sciences, and 'the problems of sex'.* Berkeley: University of California Press.

Cohen, E. (2015). Surrogacy as international business and national disgrace of Thailand. *Asian Anthropology*, *14*(2), 115–132.

Cole, M. & Stewart, K. (2014). *Our children and other animals.* Farnham: Ashgate.

Collins, C. R., Riggs, D. W. & Due, C. (2014). Constructions of the 'best interest of the child' in New South Wales parliamentary debates on surrogacy. In M. Nash (Ed.), *Reframing reproduction: Conceiving gendered experiences in late modernity* (pp. 39–53). London: Sage.

Cooper, M. (2008). *Life as surplus: Biotechnology and capitalism in the neoliberal era.* Seattle: University of Washington Press.

Cooper, M., & Waldby, C. (2014). *Clinical labor: Tissue donors and research subjects in the global bioeconomy.* Durham, NC: Duke University Press.

Cora, G. (1985). *The mother machine: Reproductive technologies from artificial insemination to artificial wombs.* New York: Harper & Row.

Crawshaw, M., Purewal, S. & Van den Akker, O. (2013). Working at the margins: The views and experiences of court social workers on Parental Orders' work in surrogacy arrangements. *British Journal of Social Work*, *43*(6), 1225–1243.

Damelio, J. & Sorenson, K. (2008). Enhancing autonomy in paid surrogacy. *Bioethics*, *5*, 269–277.

DasGupta, S. & Das Dasgupta, S. (2014). Business as usual? The violence of reproductive trafficking in the Indian context. In S. DasGupta & S. Das Dasgupta (Eds), *Globalization and transnational surrogacy in India: Outsourcing life* (pp. 179–196). New York: Lexington.

Dempsey, D. (2013). Surrogacy, gay male couples and the significance of biogenetic parenting. *New Genetics and Society*, *32*, 37–53.

Dempsey, D. (2014). Relating across international borders: Gay men forming families through overseas surrogacy. In M. C. Inhorn, W. Chavkin & J.-A. Navarro (Eds), *Globalized fatherhood* (pp. 267–290). New York: Berghahn.

Deonandan, R., Green, S. & Beinum, A. (2012). Ethical concerns for maternal surrogacy and reproductive tourism. *Journal of Medical Ethics*, *38*, 742–745.

Duggan, L. (2002). The new homonormativity: The sexual politics of neoliberalism. In R. Castronovo & D. D. Nelson (Eds), *Materializing democracy: Toward a revitalized cultural politics* (pp. 175–194). Durham, NC: Duke University Press.

Dunn, P. C., Ryan, I. J. & O'Brien, K. (1988). College students' acceptance of adoption and five alternative fertilization techniques. *Journal of Sex Research, 24*, 282–287.

Eagleton, T. (1991). *Ideology: An introduction*. London: Verso.

Evans, D. (2015). On Gawker's problem with women. Retrieved 20 May 2016, from https://medium.com/matter/on-gawker-s-problem-with-women-f1197d8c1a4e#.5kbxvr2m1.

Falk, C. (2014). *Sophia's broken crayons*. Seattle: CreateSpace Independent Publishing Platform.

Finkler, K. (2000). *Experiencing the new genetics: Family and kinship on the medical frontier*. Philadelphia: University of Pennsylvania Press.

Fisher, M. & Baum, F. (2010). The social determinants of mental health: Implications for research and health promotion. *Australian and New Zealand Journal of Psychiatry, 44*(12), 1057–1063.

Fixmer-Oraiz, N. (2013). Speaking of solidarity: Transnational gestational surrogacy and the rhetorics of reproductive (in)justice. *Frontiers, 43*, 126–163.

Foucault, M. (2003). *Society must be defended: Lectures at the College de France 1975–1976*. London: Penguin.

Franklin, S. (2001). *Dolly mixtures: The remaking of genealogy*. Durham, NC: Duke University Press.

Franklin, S. (2013). *Biological relatives: IVF, stem cells and the future of kinship*. Durham, NC: Duke University Press.

Gallagher, A. (2014). International surrogacy is dangerous and unfair. *The Sydney Morning Herald*, 5 August.

Ginsburg, F. & Rapp, R. (1991). The politics of reproduction. *Annual Review of Anthropology, 20*, 311–343.

Golombok, S., Murray, C., Jadva, V., MacCallum, F. & Lycett, E. (2004). Families created through surrogacy arrangements: Parent-child relationships in the 1st year of life. *Developmental Psychology, 40*(3), 400–411.

Gondouin, J. (2012). Adoption, surrogacy and Swedish exceptionalism. *Critical Race and Whiteness Studies, 8*(2), 1–20.

Gunnarsson Payne, J. (2016). Grammars of kinship: Biological motherhood and assisted reproduction in the age of epigenetics. *Signs: Journal of Women in Culture and Society, 41*, 483–506.

Halberstam, J. (2005). *In a queer place and time: Transgender bodies, subcultural lives*. New York: New York University Press.

Halman, L. J., Abbey, A. & Andrews, F. M. (1992). Attitudes about infertility interventions among fertile and infertile couples. *American Journal of Public Health, 82*, 191–194.

Haworth, A. (2007). Surrogate mothers: Wombs for rent. *Marie Claire*, 29 July. Retrieved 17 September 2016, from www.marieclaire.com/world-reports/news/surrogate-mothers-india.

Hays, S. (1996). *The cultural contradictions of motherhoood*. London: Yale University Press.

Herald Sun. (2011). Gay couple hit family jackpot with Indian surrogates: Two dads, four babies. 1 November, p. 4.

Hibino, Y. & Shimazono, Y. (2013). Becoming a surrogate online: 'Message board' surrogacy in Thailand. *Asian Bioethics Review, 5*(1), 56–72.

Hirschi, H. M. (2014). *Dads: A gay couple's surrogacy journey in India*. Seattle: Amazon Digital Services.

Hochschild, A. (2013). *So, how's the family? And other essays*. California: University of California Press.

Hollingworth, L. S. (1916). Social devices for impelling women to bear and rear children. *The American Journal of Sociology, 22*(1), 19–29.

Hudson, N. & Culley, L. (2011). Assisted reproductive travel: UK patient trajectories. *Reproductive Biomedicine Online, 23*, 573–581.

Imison, M. & Schweinsberg, S. (2013). Australian news media framing of medical tourism in low and middle-income countries: A content review. *BMC Public Health, 13*, 109–121.

Imrie, S. & Jadva, V. (2014). The long-term experiences of surrogates: Relationships and contact with surrogacy families in genetic and gestational surrogacy arrangements. *Reproductive Biomedicine Online, 29*, 424–435.

Inhorn, M. C. & Patrizio, P. (2009). Rethinking reproductive 'tourism' as reproductive 'exile'. *Fertility and Sterility, 92*(3), 904–906.

Inhorn, M. C. & Patrizio, P. (2012). The global landscape of cross-border reproductive care: Twenty key findings for the new millennium. *Current Opinion in Obstetrics and Gynecology, 24*, 158–163.

Jacobson, H. (2016). *Labor of love: Gestational surrogacy and the work of making babies*. New Brunswick: Rutgers University Press.

Jadva, V., Blake, L., Casey, P. & Golombok, S. (2012). Surrogacy families 10 years on: Relationship with the surrogate, decisions over disclosure and children's understanding of their surrogacy origins. *Human Reproduction*, 27, 3008–3014.

Jadva, V., Murray, C., Lycett, E., MacCallum, F. & Golombok, S. (2003). Surrogacy: The experience of surrogate mothers. *Human Reproduction, 18*, 2192–2204.

Johnson, L., Blyth, E. & Hammarberg, K. (2014). Barriers for domestic surrogacy and challenges of transnational surrogacy in the context of Australians undertaking surrogacy in India. *Journal of Law and Medicine, 22*(1), 136–154.

Jones, K. (1990). Citizenship in a woman-friendly polity. *Signs, 15*, 781–812.

Karandikar, S., Gezinski, L., Carter, J. & Kaloga, M. (2014). Economic necessity or noble cause? A qualitative study exploring motivations for gestational surrogacy in Gujarat, India. *Affilia: Journal of Women and Social Work, 29*, 224–236.

King, S. (2014). Gammy sparks call for surrogacy reform. *The Australian*, 4 August.

Kluger-Bell, K. (2013). *The very kind koala: A surrogacy story for children*. Seattle: CreateSpace Independent Publishing Platform.

Krishnan, V. (1994). Attitudes toward surrogate motherhood in Canada. *Health Care Women International, 15*, 333–357.

Kroløkke, C. (2014). Eggs and euros: A feminist perspective on reproductive travel from Denmark to Spain. *IJFAB: International Journal of Feminist Approaches to Bioethics*, 7(2), 144–163.

Kroløkke, C. H. (2015). Have eggs, will travel: The experiences and ethics of global egg donation. *Somatechnics, 5*(1), 12–31.

Kroløkke, C., Foss, K. A. & Sandoval, J. (2010). *Contemplating maternity in an era of choice: Exploration into discourses of reproduction*. Plymouth: Lexington Books.

Kroløkke, C. H. & Pant, S. (2012). 'I only need her uterus': Neo-liberal discourses on transnational surrogacy. *NORA: Nordic Journal of Feminist and Gender Research, 20*(4), 233–248.

Lambert, H. (1996). Caste, gender and locality in rural Rajasthan. In C. J. Fuller (Ed.), *Caste today* (pp. 93–123). Delhi: Oxford University Press.

Langer, B. (2002). Commodified enchantment: Children and consumer capitalism. *Thesis Eleven, 69*(1), 67–81.

Levinas, E. & Kearney, R. (1986). Dialogue with Emmanuel Levinas. In R. A. Cohen (Ed.), *Face to face with Levinas* (pp. 13–34). Albany: SUNY Press.

Lewin, E. (2009). *Gay fatherhood: Narratives of family and citizenship in America*. Chicago: University of Chicago Press.

Lewis-Long, C. (2010). *Why I'm so special: A book about surrogacy*. Bloomington: AuthorHouse.

Lewis-Long, C. (2011). *Why I'm so special: A book about surrogacy with two daddies*. Bloomington: Authorhouse.

Mamo, L. (2005). Biomedicalizing kinship: Sperm banks and the creation of affinity-ties. *Science as Culture, 14*(3), 237–264.

Mamo, L. (2007). *Queering reproduction: Achieving pregnancy in the age of technoscience*. Durham, NC: Duke University Press.

Markens, S. (2007). *Surrogate motherhood and the politics of reproduction*. Berkeley: University of California Press.

Markens, S. (2012). The global reproductive health market: U.S. media framings and public discourses about transnational surrogacy. *Social Science and Medicine, 74*, 1745–1753.

Marriner, C. (2012). When a leap of faith pays off. *Sun-Herald*, 2 September, p. 17.

Martin, A. (2007). The chimera of liberal individualism: How cells become selves in human clinical genetics. *Osiris, 22*, 205–222.

Martin, E. (1991). The egg and the sperm: How science has constructed a romance based on stereotypical male-female roles. *Signs, 16*(3), 485–501.

Martin, L. J. (2015). *Reproductive tourism in the United States: Creating family in the mother country*. New York: Routledge.

Maushart, S. (1997). *The mask of motherhood*. Sydney: Random house Press.

May, A. & Tenzek, K. (2011). Seeking Mrs. Right: Uncertainty reduction in online surrogacy ads. *Qualitative Research Reports in Communication, 12*(1), 27–33.

May, A. & Tenzek, K. (2016). 'A gift we are unable to create ourselves': Uncertainty reduction in online classified ads posted by gay men pursuing surrogacy. *Journal of GLBT Family Studies*, 1–22.

Menichiello, M. (2012). *A gay couple's journey through surrogacy: Intended fathers*. New York: Haworth Press.

Millbank, J. (2012). From Alice and Evelyn to Isabella: Exploring the narrative and norms of 'new' surrogacy in Australia. *Griffith Law Review, 21*(1), 101–136.

Murdoch, L. (2014). Australian couple leaves Down syndrome baby with Thai surrogate. *The Sydney Morning Herald*, 1 August.

Murphy, D. (2015). *Gay men pursuing parenthood through surrogacy: Reconfiguring kinship*. Sydney: UNSW Press.

Murray, M. (Ed.). (2014). *Critical health psychology*. Basingstoke: Palgrave Macmillan.

Nash, C. (2015). *Genetic geographies: The trouble with ancestry*. Minneapolis: University of Minnesota Press.

Nathanson, J. & Tuley, L. C. (2009). *Mother knows best: Talking back to the 'experts'*. Toronto: Demeter Press.

Nelkin, D. & Lindee, M. S. (2004). *The DNA mystique: The gene as a cultural icon*. Ann Arbor: University of Michigan Press.

Nicoll, F. (2000). Indigenous sovereignty and the violence of perspective: A white woman's coming out story. *Australian Feminist Studies, 15*(33), 369–386.

O'Flaherty, C. & O'Flaherty, N. (2012). *Baby Ava: An Irish surrogacy story*. Dublin: Liberties Press.

Orloff, A. (1993). Gender and the social rights of citizenship: The comparative analysis of gender relations and welfare states. *American Sociological Review, 58*(3), 303–328.

Palattiyil, G., Blyth, E., Sidhva, D. & Balakrishnan, G. (2010). Globalization and cross border reproductive services: Ethical implications of surrogacy in India for social work. *International Social Work, 53*(5), 686–700.

Pande, A. (2009). 'It may be her eggs but it's my blood': Surrogates and everyday forms of kinship in India. *Qualitative Sociology, 32*(4), 379–397.

Pande, A. (2010). Commercial surrogacy in India: Manufacturing a perfect mother-worker. *Signs, 35*(4), 969–992.

Pande, A. (2011). Transnational commercial surrogacy in India: Gifts for global sisters? *Reproductive Biomedicine Online, 23*(5), 618–625.

Phillips Pellet, S. (2006). *The kangaroo pouch: A story about surrogacy for young children*. Berkeley: Haven Stone Media.

Poote, A. & Van den Akker, O. (2009). British women's attitudes to surrogacy. *Human Reproduction, 24*(1), 139–145.

Ragoné, H. (1994). *Surrogate motherhood: Conception in the heart*. Boulder: Westview Press.

Ragoné, H. (1996). Chasing the blood tie: Surrogate mothers, adoptive mothers and fathers. *American Ethnologist, 23*(2), 352–365.

Ragoné, H. (1999). The gift of life: Surrogate motherhood, gamete donation, and constructions of altruism. In L. L. Layne (Ed.), *Transformative motherhood: On giving and getting in a consumer culture* (pp. 65–88). New York: New York University Press.

Raymond, J. R. (1993). *Women as wombs: Reproductive technologies and the battle over women's freedom*. San Francisco: Harper.

Readings, J., Blake, L., Casey, P., Jadva, V. & Golombok, S. (2011). Secrecy, disclosure and everything in-between: Decisions of parents of children conceived by donor insemination, egg donation and surrogacy. *Reproductive Biomedicine Online, 22*(5), 485–495.

Ressler, I., Jaeger, A. & Lindheim, S. (2012). Evolving ethical issues in third party reproduction: Local and global considerations. *World Journal of Medical Genetics, 2*(1), 1–8.

Richards, B. (2015). 'Can I take the normal one?': Unrelated commercial surrogacy and child abandonment. *Hofstra Law Review, 44*(1), 201–235.

Richards, G. (2003). *Race, racism and psychology: Towards a reflexive history*. New York: Routledge.

Riggs, D. W. (2005). Locating control: Psychology and the cultural production of 'healthy subject positions'. *Culture, Health & Sexuality, 9*, 87–100.

Riggs, D. W. (2009). Race privilege and its role in the 'disappearance' of birth families and adoptive children in debates over adoption by non-heterosexual people in Australia. In D. Cuthbert & C. Spark (Eds), *Other people's children: Adoption in Australia* (pp. 161–175). Melbourne: Australian Scholarly Publishing.

Riggs, D. W. (2013). Transgender men's self-representations of bearing children post-transition. In F. Green & M. Friedman (Eds), *Chasing rainbows* (pp. 62–71). Toronto: Demeter Press.

Riggs, D. W. (2014). What makes a man? Thomas Beattie, embodiment, and 'mundane transphobia'. *Feminism and Psychology, 24*, 157–171.

Riggs, D. W. (2015a). *Pink herrings: Fantasy, object choice, and sexuation*. London: Karnac.

Riggs, D. W. (2015b). '25 degrees of separation' versus the 'ease of doing it closer to home': Motivations to offshore surrogacy arrangements amongst Australian citizens. *Somatechnics, 5*, 52–68.

Riggs, D. W. & Bartholomaeus, C. (2016). The desire for a child amongst a sample of heterosexual Australian couples. *Journal of Reproductive and Infant Psychology, 34*, 442–450.

Riggs, D. W. & Bartholomaeus, C. (2017). 'It's just what you do': Australian middle class heterosexual couples negotiating compulsory parenthood. *Feminism & Psychology*. Online First. doi: 10.1177/0959353516675637.

Riggs, D. W., Delfabbro, P. H. & Augoustinos, M. (2009). Negotiating foster families: Identification and desire. *British Journal of Social Work, 39*, 789–806.

Riggs, D. W. & Dempsey, D. (2015). Gay men's narratives of pregnancy in the context of commercial surrogacy. In N. Burton (Ed.), *Birth and its meanings: Representations of pregnancy, childbirth and parenting* (pp. 73–87). Toronto: Demeter Press.

Riggs, D. W. & Due, C. (2010). Gay men, race privilege, and surrogacy in India. *Outskirts: Feminisms Along the Edge, 22*. Retrieved 19 June 2017, from www.outskirts.arts.uwa.edu.au/volumes/volume-22/riggs.

Riggs, D. W. & Due, C. (2012). Representations of surrogacy in submissions to a parliamentary inquiry in New South Wales. *Techne, 16*, 71–84.

Riggs, D. W. & Due, C. (2013). Representations of reproductive citizenship and vulnerability in media reports of offshore surrogacy. *Citizenship Studies, 17*, 956–969.

Riggs, D. W., Due, C. & Power, J. (2015). Gay men's experiences of surrogacy clinics in India. *Journal of Family Planning and Reproductive Health, 41*, 48–53.

Riggs, D. W. & Peel, E. (2016). *Critical kinship studies: An introduction to the field*. Basingstoke: Palgrave Macmillan.

Roach Anleu, S. (1992). Surrogacy: For love but not for money? *Gender & Society, 6*, 30–48.

Roberts, D. (1997). *Killing the black body: Race, reproduction, and the meaning of liberty*. New York: Pantheon Books.

Roberts, D. (2002). Shattered bonds: The color of child welfare. *Children and Youth Services Review, 24*(11), 877–880.

Robertson, C. (2009). *Legislation on altruistic surrogacy in NSW*. Sydney: New South Wales Parliamentary Library.

Rollin, B. (1974). Motherhood: Need or myth? In E. Peck & J. Senderowitz (Eds), *Pronatalism: The myth of mom and apple pie* (pp. 149–150). New York: Thomas Y. Crowell Company.

Rotabi, K. & Bromfield, N. (2012). The decline of intercountry adoptions and new practices of global surrogacy: Global exploitation and human rights concerns. *Affilia: Journal of Women and Social Work, 27*(2), 129–141.

Rothman, B. (1989). *Recreating motherhood: Ideology and technology in a patriarchal society*. New York: W.W. Norton.

Rubin, G. (1975). The traffic in women: Notes on the 'political economy' of sex. In R. R. Reiter (Ed.), *Toward an anthropology of women* (pp. 157–210). New York: Monthly Review Press.

Rudrappa, S. (2010). Making India the 'mother destination': Outsourcing labor to Indian surrogates. *Research in the Sociology of Work, 20*, 253–285.

Rudrappa, S. (2014). Conceiving fatherhood: Gay men and Indian surrogate mothers. In M. C. Inhorn, W. Chavkin & J.-A. Navarro (Eds), *Globalized fatherhood* (pp. 291–311). New York: Berghahn.

Rudrappa, S. (2015). *Discounted life: The price of global surrogacy in India*. New York: New York University Press.

Rudrappa, S. & Collins, C. (2015). Altruistic agencies and compassionate consumers: Moral framing of transnational surrogacy. *Gender & Society, 29*, 937–959.

Sartre, J.-P. (1976). *Critique of dialectical reason*. Trans. Alan Sheridan Smith, Ed. Jonathon Ree. London: New Left Books.

Schneider, D. M. (1968). *American kinship: A cultural account*. Chicago: University of Chicago Press.

Schneider, D. M. (1984). *A critique of the study of kinship*. Michigan: University of Michigan Press.

Scholz, B. & Riggs, D. W. (2014). Sperm donors' account of lesbian recipients: Heterosexualisation as a tool for warranting claims to children's 'best interests'. *Psychology and Sexuality, 5*, 247–257.

Shalev, S. & Lemish, D. (2011). Women as consumers of reproductive technology: Media representation versus reality. *Journal of Interdisciplinary Feminist Thought, 5*, 1–23.

Sharp, L. A. (2000). The commodification of the body and its parts. *Annual Review of Anthropology, 29*, 287–328.

Speier, A. R. (2011). Brokers, consumers and the internet: How North American consumers navigate their infertility journeys. *Reproductive Biomedicine Online, 23*(5), 592–599.

Stainton Rogers, W. (1991). *Explaining health and illness: An exploration of diversity*. Hertfordshire: Harvester Wheatsheaf.

Strathern, M. (1988). *The gender of the gift: Problems with women and problems with society in Melanesia*. Berkeley: University of California Press.

Strathern, M. (1992). *Reproducing the future: Anthropology, kinship, and the new reproductive technologies*. Manchester: Manchester University Press.

Strathern, M. (2003). Still giving nature a helping hand? Surrogacy: A debate about technology and society. In R. Cook, S. Day Sclater & F. Kaganas (Eds), *Surrogate motherhood: International perspectives* (pp. 281–296). Oxford: Hart Publishing.

Suzuki, K., Hoshi, K., Minai, J., Yanaihara, T., Takeda, Y. & Yamagata, Z. (2006). Analysis of national representative opinion surveys concerning gestational surrogacy in Japan. *European Journal of Obstetrics & Gynecology Reproductive Biology, 126*, 39–47.

Teman, E. (2010). *Birthing a mother: The surrogate body and the pregnant self.* Berkeley: University of California Press.

Thompson, C. (2005). *Making parents: The ontological choreography of reproductive technologies*. Cambridge, MA: MIT Press.

Turner, B. S. (2001). The erosion of citizenship. *The British Journal of Sociology, 52*(2), 189–209.

Van den Akker, O. (2003). Genetic and gestational surrogate mothers' experience of surrogacy. *Journal of Reproductive and Infant Psychology, 21*(2), 145–161.

Van den Akker, O., Camara, I. & Hunt, B. (2016). 'Together … for only a moment': British newspaper constructions of altruistic non-commercial surrogate mothers. *Journal of Reproductive and Infant Psychology, 34*(3), 271–281.

Van Reyk, P. (2007). Baby love: Gay donor father narratives of intimacy. *Gay and Lesbian Issues and Psychology Review, 3*(1), 44–52.

Vora, K. (2009). Indian transnational surrogacy and the commodification of vital energy. *Subjectivity, 28*(1), 266–278.

Vora, K. (2010). Medicine, markets and the pregnant body: Indian commercial surrogacy and reproductive labor in a transnational frame. *Scholar and Feminist Online, 9*(1/2). Retrieved 19 June 2017, from http://sfonline.barnard.edu/reprotech/vora_01.htm.

Vora, K. (2014). Experimental sociality and gestational surrogacy in the Indian ART clinic. *Ethnos: Journal of Anthropology, 79*, 63–83.

Vora, K. (2015). *Life support: Biocapital and the new history of outsourced labor*. Minneapolis: University of Minnesota Press.

Warner, J. (2013). *The journey of same-sex surrogacy: Discovering ultimate joy*. Tennessee: Zygote Publishing.

Weston, K. (1990). *Families we choose: Lesbians, gays, kinship*. New York: Columbia University Press.

Westoby, Richard. (2013). *Our 'journey': One couple's guide to US surrogacy*. Seattle: Amazon Digital Services.

Whittaker, A. (2011). Cross-border assisted reproduction care in Asia: Implications for access, equity and regulations. *Reproductive Health Matters, 19*(37), 107–116.

Whittaker, A. (2014). Merit and money: The situated ethics of transnational commercial surrogacy in Thailand. *International Journal of Feminist Approaches to Bioethics,* 7(2), 100–120.

Whittaker, A. (2015) Technology, biopolitics, rationalities and choices: Recent studies of reproduction. *Medical Anthropology*, *34*(3), 259–273.

Whittaker, A. & Speier, A. (2010). 'Cycling overseas': Care, commodification, and stratification in cross-border reproductive travel. *Medical Anthropology*, *29*(4), 363–383.

Young, I. M. (1994). Gender as seriality: Thinking about women as a social collective. *Signs*, *19*, 713–738.

Zelizer, V. A. (1994). *Pricing the priceless child: The changing social value of children*. New Jersey: Princeton University Press.

Zelizer, V. A. (2005). *The purchase of intimacy*. New Jersey: Princeton University Press.

INDEX